Practical Issues in Anesthesia and Intensive Care

W0050721

Biagio Allaria
Editor

Practical Issues
in Anesthesia
and Intensive Care

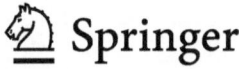 Springer

Editor
Biagio Allaria
Past Director of Critical Care Department
Istituto Nazionale per lo Studio e la Cura dei Tumori
National Cancer Institute
Milan, Italy

This is the English version of the Italian edition published under the title
Excerpta Anestesiologica – Volume 1, edited by Biagio Allaria
© Springer-Verlag Italia 2011

Translation: Jonathan C. Spurrell and Ludovica Arcelli Betts
The translation of this work has been funded by SEPS
Segretariato Europeo per le Pubblicazioni Scientifiche

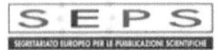 Via Val d'Aposa 7, 40123 Bologna, Italy
seps@seps.it - www.seps.it

ISBN 978-88-470-2459-5   ISBN 978-88-470-2460-1 (eBook)

DOI 10.1007/978-88-470-2460-1

Springer Milan Dordrecht Heidelberg London New York

Library of Congress Control Number: 2011940269

© Springer-Verlag Italia 2012

This work is subject to copyright. All rights are reserved by the Publisher, whether the whole or part of the material is concerned, specifically the rights of translation, reprinting, reuse of illustrations, recitation, broadcasting, reproduction on microfilms or in any other physical way, and transmission or information storage and retrieval, electronic adaptation, computer software, or by similar or dissimilar methodology now known or hereafter developed. Exempted from this legal reservation are brief excerpts in connection with reviews or scholarly analysis or material supplied specifically for the purpose of being entered and executed on a computer system, for exclusive use by the purchaser of the work. Duplication of this publication or parts thereof is permitted only under the provisions of the Copyright Law of the Publisher's location, in its current version, and permission for use must always be obtained from Springer. Permissions for use may be obtained through RightsLink at the Copyright Clearance Center. Violations are liable to prosecution under the respective Copyright Law.

The use of general descriptive names, registered names, trademarks, service marks, etc. in this publication does not imply , even in the absence of a specific statement, that such names are exempt from the relevant protective laws and regulations and therefore free for general use.

While the advice and information in this book are believed to be true and accurate at the date of publication, neither the authors nor the editors nor the publisher can accept any legal responsibility for any errors or omissions that may be made. The publisher makes no warranty, express or implied, with respect to the material contained herein.

7 6 5 4 3 2 1   2012 2013 2014

Cover design: Ikona S.r.l., Milan, Italy
Typesetting: Graphostudio, Milan, Italy

Springer-Verlag Italia S.r.l. – Via Decembrio 28 – I-20137 Milan
Springer is a part of Springer Science+Business Media (www.springer.com)

Preface

For specialists whose work involves caring for critical patients, it is particularly useful to assess matters that are of considerable interest in the management of such patients, where clear ideas and the ability to make important decisions quickly are necessary.

These assessments must be up-to-date and concise, and include clear and useful messages for clinical practice.

This has been our aim in compiling this easy-to-read work, with each question being addressed by an expert in that field, and with an assessment of the latest developments.

The material used to compile this book is taken from recent works that are arranged every year by *Medical Evidence Italia* for those who work in the fields of anaesthesia and resuscitation.

Medical Evidence Italia produces accredited updates for the Italian Ministry of Health. We would like to express our thanks to the Ministry, along with all the authors who have contributed to this book, Springer, who came up with the idea, and Jonathan C. Spurrell and Ludovica Arcelli Betts, who have translated it.

Milan, December 2011   Biagio Allaria

Contents

**7   Hypercapnic Acidosis in Protective Mechanical Ventilation
(a Tolerated Compromise or Another Means of Protection?)**   93
Biagio Allaria

8   Are We Sure We Are Using Drugs Correctly in Critical Patients? .. 107
Biagio Allaria

**9   The Problem of Decontamination of the Digestive Tract
and Gastric Acid Suppression in Intensive Care** 121
Biagio Allaria

**10   Renal, Cardiac and Pulmonary Involvement in Patients with
Supraventricular Tachycardia: a Typical Holistic Vision by
an Intensive Care Physician** 135
Biagio Allaria

Contributors

Biagio Allaria Past Director of Critical Care Department, Istituto Nazionale per lo Studio e la Cura dei Tumori - National Cancer Institute, Milan, Italy

Patrizia Andreoni 2nd Anesthesia and Critical Care Service, Transplant Department, Ospedale Niguarda Ca' Granda, Milan, Italy

Emanuela Biagioni Department of Anesthesia and Intensive Care, University Hospital of Modena, Modena, Italy

Davide Chiumello Department of Anesthesiology, Resuscitation and Pain Medicine, Fondazione IRCCS Ca' Granda Ospedale Maggiore Policlinico, Milan, Italy

Stefania Colombo 2nd Anesthesia and Critical Care Service, Transplant Department, Ospedale Niguarda Ca' Granda, Milan, Italy

Paola Cozzi 2nd Anesthesia and Critical Care Service, Transplant Department, Ospedale Niguarda Ca' Granda, Milan, Italy

Andrea De Gasperi 2nd Anesthesia and Critical Care Service, Transplant Department, Ospedale Niguarda Ca' Granda, Milan, Italy

Marco Dei Poli Emergency, Critical Care and First Aid, IRCCS Policlinico San Donato, San Donato Milanese (MI), Italy

Tommaso Fossali Department of Anesthesiology, Resuscitation and Pain Medicine, Fondazione IRCCS Ca' Granda Ospedale Maggiore Policlinico, Milan, Italy

Massimo Girardis Department of Anesthesia and Intensive Care, University Hospital of Modena, Modena, Italy

Silvia Gramaticopolo Anesthesiology and Resuscitation Department, Local Health Unit ULSS 6, Vicenza, Italy

Marco Marietta Department of Oncology and Haematology, University of Modena and Reggio Emilia, Modena, Italy

Ernestina Mazza 2nd Anesthesia and Critical Care Service, Transplant Department, Ospedale Niguarda Ca' Granda, Milan, Italy

Pasquale Piccinni Head of Anesthesiology and Resuscitation Department, Local Health Unit ULSS 6, Vicenza, Italy

Marco Resta Emergency, Critical Care and First Aid, IRCCS Policlinico San Donato, San Donato Milanese (MI), Italy

Sara Sher Department of Anesthesiology, Resuscitation and Pain Medicine, Fondazione IRCCS Ca' Granda Ospedale Maggiore Policlinico, Milan, Italy

Intensive Care for Elderly Patients: Clinical, Ethical and Economic Considerations

Marco Dei Poli and Marco Resta

1.1   Introduction

Nearly every work on the issues surrounding intensive care for elderly patients starts out with the same premise: that in the western world the future is likely to bring a shortage of young people and an increasing number of over-80s.

The second premise is the growing impact of the elderly population on social, healthcare and pension systems, and on the need for an ethical justification of expenditure that is based on finite resources.

The third point is to identify prognosis markers that influence the admission to or refusal of more complex and costlier treatment, as well as the point at which treatment is withheld or withdrawn, taking into account the wishes of the patient and his or her family.

It is useful for us to begin with this premise, too. If, on the one hand, population aging is the result of improved living conditions in our society (referring to the western, or industrialised, world), there is, on the other hand, an urgent need for every country to bring its social and healthcare systems under control. In Italy at the moment, 20% of the population is over 65, compared to the European average of 15.7%. Eurostat predicts that within 50 years Italy's elderly will account for 33.4% of the total population. In terms of the very elderly (or the "oldest old", as the Americans say), Italy has the highest rate in Europe, with 3.9% of the overall population belonging to this category.

In biological and medical terms, an elderly person is someone who has reached a specified age, usually around 60 years. The end of adulthood marks the beginning of old age, followed by very old age (over 80 years) and then death. The most useful classification is that of *young old* (65-75 years), followed

M. Dei Poli (✉)
Emergency, Critical Care and First Aid
IRCCS Policlinico San Donato, San Donato Milanese (MI), Italy
e-mail: deipolimd@gmail.com

Biagio Allaria (ed.), *Practical Issues in Anesthesia and Intensive Care*
© Springer-Verlag Italia 2012

by *old old* (between 75-80 years and 85-90 years) and *oldest old* (85-90 years or more). The descriptions "survival beyond life expectancy at birth" and "life expectancy without disability" are equally useful.

But even these descriptions, even when adjusted, are essentially limited. We know from daily experience that age itself is rarely a reflection of the aging process. For example, a 40-year-old may be considered "old" because of heart and circulation problems while a 70-year-old may, on the other hand, have a "young" heart and arteries despite the obvious signs of aging. The elderly person may have retained a substantial amount of physical energy, and it is often the case that good memory, concentration, logic and creativity go hand in hand with the physical appearance of an old person as a result of advanced aging. However, there are those who, as well as maintaining relatively young physical character-istics, show the distressing signs of mental aging with short-term memory loss, impaired concentration, etc. These examples show that physical, or biological, aging often does not reflect psychological aging, and that making clear distinc-tions between the different stages of life, particularly aging and old age, is not only inappropriate but also leads to prejudice.

These concepts converge in the word "fragility", which is commonly used in gerontology to imply vulnerability to adverse events, with "fragile" having a worse outcome than "non fragile" in patients with a similar same state of health receiving the same care.

Furthermore, as previously stated, a so-called "demographic transition" is underway in the world, characterised by a drop in fertility and a corresponding reduction in mortality rates, especially among the elderly. The chances of sur-viving longer into old age are higher, leading to a relative swell in the number of elderly people, at an annual growth rate of 2%, which is higher than the over-all population growth rate. This trend is expected to continue for at least 25 years.

Hospitalisation of elderly patients for acute diseases is on the rise, as is the demand for access to intensive care. In Europe, as in the United States of America, intensive care for elderly patients is the subject of much debate as well as a cause for concern. In Italy, the GiViTi database compiled by the Mario Negri Institute (Margherita II project) calculated an admission rate of 31.5% in 2006 for intensive care in over 75s for a total of 46,401 admissions. This rate was almost identical to admission rates for medical reasons (33.1%), elective surgery (31.9%) or emergency surgery (31.3%).

Most of the literature tends to regard old age as 80 years and over, but often the age limit for intensive care is considered to be 85.

Various issues arise in the wide-ranging debate on intensive care for elderly patients. The first issue concerns the decisions made during triage as to whether or not to admit a patient to intensive care. The second involves the admissions procedure, which often depends on length of time the patient is expected to stay in hospital, the use of resources and discharge procedures. The third issue con-cerns long-term success after intensive care in terms of death, quality of life and autonomy.

1.2   Admissions Criteria

It is understandable that the elderly, including the over 80s, should have greater access to intensive care [1]. Each day doctors working in ICUs (*intensive care units*) must make difficult decisions about who should be given rare, specialist beds and who should be refused. This is the process of triage. There are many reasons and circumstances for these decisions, which include the request for admission, followed by an assessment of the severity of the disease as well as an assessment of the number of beds available [2].

Triage is based on a probability assessment of the disease outcome, the expected effect of treatment on the disease, the predicted relationship between the benefit of treatment and the suffering involved for the patient and his or her family, and the social cost of treatment. The ethical and religious views of everybody involved are also taken into consideration, often without all the information that would ideally be required for triage.

Very few studies have been conducted on the triage process for over 80s in intensive care [3]. An analysis of studies into admissions and refusals for intensive care in all age brackets shows that the refusal rate varies greatly, from 23% to 72%. Factors associated with refusal of admission were advanced aged, significant comorbidity or pre-existing disabilities. The refusal rate in these cases was 72%.

Other studies show that only advanced age is a risk factor for death in intensive care [4]. Numerical age alone, however, would not be the sole reason for refusing to admit an elderly patient to an ICU, since there are many cases of favourable outcomes and a good quality of life after discharge [5]. Furthermore, it is interesting to note that the outcome of long-term care in elderly patients is affected more by pre-existing and underlying disorders that by age. This accounts for the growing availability of treatment for elderly patients in intensive care.

It has, however, been shown that the elderly, once admitted to intensive care, do in fact receive less care (mechanical ventilation, CRRT) than younger patients, once a statistical adjustment has been made for the severity of the disease [6]. It is also clear that the increase in admission rates for elderly patients in intensive care has not been matched by a similar willingness to provide intensive treatment. This is due to the potential harmful effects of radical treatment approaches, fear of failure and financial restrictions.

Nevertheless, it can be said that technological advancements and social progress have improved conditions for the admission of the oldest old to intensive care. Who, therefore, should we admit to ICUs, and which cases should be discussed?

It is easy to explain to those who, like the patient's family, do not spend every day in the ICU that the methods used in intensive care are a double-edged sword. It is clear from the now mandatory and widespread use of analgesia that a great deal of pain is often experienced in ICUs. Everyone can see that the artificial maintenance of vital functions may be nothing more than a temporary step towards increased autonomy for the patient.

Amongst other things, separation from loved ones, promiscuity and sometimes a conscious inability to communicate are evident and can be fully justified in young patients or in the event of unforeseen postoperative complications. But in the oldest old, in whom there is some uncertainty, these factors turn into a series of difficult questions regarding treatment. The problem is intensified when access to intensive care is requested by elderly patients with a poor short-term prognosis for related diseases (such as surgery-resistant or chemotherapy-resistant tumours, malignant tumours with a prognosis of under 12 months, or non-reversible, advanced, chronic organ failure), or when it is requested by immunodepressed patients, those with cachexia as a result of chronic malnutrition, or those with very advanced cognitive-behavioural disorders. It is very common for experienced care providers (internists, oncologists, endocrinologists, nephrologists) to base their judgements only on their area of expertise, often giving a favourable opinion regarding a patient's outcome based on the disease in question whilst failing to contemplate his or her overall condition and age. The concept of triage, especially in Italian culture, is often forgotten faced with the opportunity of admitting a patient to intensive care, often prompted by extensive medical technology and the "non-culture" of death.

As well as the provision of more space for geriatric patients, we shall discuss the reasonable use of resources and treatment approaches, a clear and coherent admissions protocol, full transparency with the patient's family and with other specialists, the use of objective criteria to assess the patient's prospects, the course, the time at which to alter the treatment approach, and above all a mature attitude regarding end-of-life care and the reduction of suffering.

1.3 Outcome

There must be a clear starting point when discussing the influence of age on outcome, in order to correctly understand the works that have been published on the subject.

Since intensive care for elderly patients is often postponed, those with the highest comorbidity can be underrepresented in case reports, leading to an excessively favourable view of the effect that age has on mortality rates [7]. However, the decision to withdraw or not to initiate aggressive treatment can lead to increased mortality in elderly patients, to whom this practice is more commonly applied.

Based on these premises, though, it seems reasonable enough to suppose that there is a relationship between old age (the *oldest old*) and favourable outcomes in intensive care. In a 1995 study [8] it was shown that the mortality rate in one hospital for patients with mechanical ventilation was 70% among the over-80s compared to 32% in patients aged less than 30 years.

Prematurely discharging elderly patients from ICUs may result in higher readmission rates, as demonstrated in a multicenter study in 30 ICUs in Austria [9].

Data from the SUPPORT study [10] show that the risk of death during a stay in an ICU increases by 1% per year from the age of 16 to 70, but by 2% per year after 70. In the Dutch NICE study [11] the death rate for over 85 year olds in hospital was four times higher than for patients aged under 65.

It may therefore be thought that it is rational to restrict the admission of over 80s to intensive care or even to limit treatment. To complicate the problem and prevent hasty conclusions, numerous studies based on multivariate analyses [12] show that age is not an independent predictor of mortality, and it is worth mentioning that not all octogenarians admitted for intensive care are lost causes. What, therefore, are the factors that affect the prediction of survival or death in this type of patient?

As stated above, assessments of outcome will be analysed based on a range of works available in the literature using the following criteria: intensive care length of stay (ICU LOS), hospital length of stay (Hospital LOS), type of severity score and points awarded (APACHE, II, SAPS II, etc.), ventilation rate, extent of intensive care according to type of care and number of points (TISS, NEMS, Omega), ICU mortality rate, hospital mortality rate, and long-term mortality rate with various follow-up periods (3 months, 1 year, etc.).

In various studies, the diagnosis on admission is a key factor when predicting the outcome. For example, the mortality rate for patients aged between 80 and 84 years who were diagnosed with an infection on admission to hospital is 85%, compared to 58% for patients in the same age bracket who had gastrointestinal disorders [8].

Treatment success for geriatric patients admitted with head injuries is known to be half that of younger patients in terms of mortality and brain function [13]. In a Dutch study of elderly patients receiving elective and emergency surgery [14], the survival rate is similar to that observed in the general population for elective surgery, whilst for emergency surgery the mortality rate after one year is about 65%.

Similar data emerge from a Spanish study [15] which assessed events following intensive care, i.e. in Intermediate Care Units (IMCUs), in which short-term mortality was correctly predicted based on the seriousness of the disease on admission and the extent of intensive care, while comorbidity mainly had an effect on mortality after one year. The age brackets used for these elderly patients were relevant only for long-term mortality.

The role of comorbidity has been widely explored in an attempt to identify accurate predictors of treatment success. Comorbidity is the overall effect of diseases that are unrelated to the main diagnosis on admission, but which contribute to the clinical outcome and economic consequences (use of resources, functional status on discharge and length of hospitalisation). Curiously, although it would be easy to imagine the potentially long list of major comorbidities seen in elderly patients on admission to ICUs, no studies are available that specifically cover the over 80s.

In studies conducted in patients who were not selected according to age, it is easy to observe that comorbidity is taken into account with the APACHE II and

III points systems, but not with SAPS II or the MPM (Mortality Probability Model). In these studies, the status of the chronic disease prior to admission to an ICU did not affect mortality, but the points system was a good overall predictor [16].

Other factors affecting the outcome of intensive care for elderly patients are malnutrition (expressed as baseline BMI (body mass index) and often diagnosed by internists, leading to delays in the restoration of bodily functions and a greater need for care at home [17]), delirium as a predictor of reintubation, prolonged hospitalisation and death [18]. Further complications that may influence prognosis include serious adverse drug reactions, hospital-acquired infections and bedsores [19].

1.4 Residual Quality of Life, Disability on Admission and Discharge

As with comorbidity, it has been suggested that the level of dependence (or rather the level of disability) may be associated with a worse prognosis on discharge from intensive care, leading to a debate on the use prognosis markers. In 2005 only 16 studies (conducted over a 13-year period) were available on the assessment of autonomy and residual quality of life following the admission of elderly patients to intensive care. In 1991 Mayer Oakes [20] showed that among the elderly survivors of treatment in ICUs, the number of entirely dependent patients was considerably lower than the number of non-survivors. In a more recent work [19] the prognosis of elderly patients in ICUs depended not only on the APACHE II score on admission, but also on the extent to which functional independence had been lost as well as the presence of cognitive impairment on admission. The ADL (activities of daily living) score has proved useful in this respect (Table 1.1).

Disability and comorbidity prior to the start of intensive care are both danger signs: this is confirmed by the fact that the peak mortality rate for the oldest old is three months after discharge from ICU [21].

Still more remarkable, however, is the assessment of disability symptoms on discharge from hospital in patients who have spent time in critical care: a much greater level of dependence may reduce quality of life to what would probably have been too low for admission in the first place. An example of this is a cohort of elderly patients without dementia for whom hospitalisation for a critical disease increased the risk of debilitating cognitive impairment in contrast with a control group that was not admitted to hospital [22]. In reality, in a 2005 review by Hennessy et al. [23] involving 3,347 patients from 16 studies, HRQOL (health-related quality of life) and functional status in elderly patients who survived intensive care is moderate, even if ADL independence in the various subgroups was considerably reduced in patients who stayed in ICUs for more than 30 days, as it was in those who stayed for more than 5 days.

There is undoubtedly a problem with the methods used to assess patient ability and quality of life. Regardless of any other considerations, excessive empha-

Table 1.1 ADL Point

Activity	Independence 1 point	Dependence 0 points
	No supervision, direction or personal assistance	With supervision, direction, personal assistance or total care
Bathing	Bathes self completely or needs help in bathing only a single part of the body such as the back, genital area or disabled extremity	Needs help with bathing more than one part of the body, getting in or out of the tub or shower. Requires total bathing
Dressing	Gets clothes from closets and drawers and puts on clothes and garments complete with fasteners. May have help tying shoes	Needs help with dressing self or needs to be completely dressed
Toileting	Goes to toilet, gets on and off, arranges clothes, cleans genital area without help	Needs help transferring to toilet, cleaning self or uses bedpan or commode
Transferring	Moves in and out of bed or chair unassisted. Mechanical transferring aids are acceptable	Needs help in moving from bed to chair or requires a complete transfer
Continence	Exercises complete self control over urination and defecation	Is partially or totally incontinent of bowel or bladder
Feeding	Gets food from plate into mouth without help. Preparation of food may be done by another person	Needs partial or total help with feeding or requires parenteral feeding

The table contains a series of activities that identify the level of autonomy of a patient. Points vary from 6 (complete autonomy) to 0 (complete dependence with total dependence in daily life).

sis on physical ability may underestimate the acceptance level for limitations in elderly patients who may in turn consider their affective and cognitive abilities to be moderately good.

Of the 1,266 patients aged over 80 included in the Hospitalized Elderly Longitudinal Project, very few said they would want to swap a longer life with varying degrees of disability for a shorter life of perfect health. In the study by Garrouste Orgeas [3] in a cohort of 180 over-80s, half stated that they did not want to be admitted to intensive care. In reality, autonomy did not deteriorate after admission, but in 60% of the survivors (50% of the 180 patients admitted) who were transferred to intermediate care facilities, quality of life (QOL) was decidedly worse than levels reported in previous studies.

Where care was withheld from a patient because of a bad prognosis based on mental performance on admission, it was seen that no prognosis markers had yet been made available to doctors and nurses [24]. Even with many limitations and areas for further discussion, it is currently only possible to use indexes that have already been authorised for rehabilitation facilities, but which are not appropriate for intensive care. Two of the most common indexes are included (Tables 1.2 and 1.3).

It is hoped that in future there will be many more contributions to this crucial debate in the literature, since intensive care patients and major users of resources are always most deeply involved.

Table 1.2 LODS[a]

Neurologic system
Glasgow Coma Score
Nervous system overall score
Cardiovascular system
Heart rate (beats/min)
Systolic blood pressure (mmHg)
Cardiovascular system overall score
Renal system
Serum urea nitrogen
Creatinine
Urine output (L/day)
Renal system overall score
Pulmonary system
PaO_2 (mmHg)/FiO_2 or PaO_2 [kPa]/FiO_2
Pulmonary system overall score
Haematologic system
White blood cell count (10^9/L)
Platelets (10^9/L)
Haematologic system overall score
Hepatic system
Bilirubin
Prothrombin
Hepatic system overall score
Total LODS score
Probability of death (%)

[a] Logistic Organ Dysfunction System.
The table contains various terms related to various organs. For each organ, an assessment is requested that can be linked to the results of blood chemistry tests or results from clinical tests. Assessments are given a numerical value of 0 to 5, which in turn generates points that are summarised after the words "name of organ overall score". The *sum of these points* makes a LODS score of between 0 (normal patient) and 22, which corresponds to a patient with very serious multiple organ dysfunction. The *individual points*, however, are inserted into a programme that can estimate the mortality rate.
Automatic counters can be found online using the following links:
http://www.sfar.org/scores2/lods2.html
http://statpages.org/lods.html

1.5   Outcome Markers

The English-speaking medical world clearly invites us to take a more rational and less emotional approach, balancing probability assessments with more serious considerations of prospects and the possibility of experiencing the improbable.

Table 1.3 Barthel disability index

1. Feeding	0 = unable; 5 = needs help (e.g., cutting food); 10 = independent
2. Bathing	0 = dependent; 5 = independent
3. Grooming	0 = needs help; 5 = independent face/hair/teeth/shaving (inserts blade if using razor)
4. Dressing	0 = dependent; 5 = needs help but can do about half unaided in reasonable time; 10 = independent (including buttons, zips, laces)
5. Bowels	0 = incontinent; 5 = occasional incident or needs help; 10 = continent
6. Bladder	0 = dependent; 5= needs some help with balance, dressing/undressing or using toilet paper 10= independent use of toilet or bedpan
7. Toilet use	0 = incapable, no balance when seated;
8. Transfers	5 = able to sit down, but needs maximum assistance transferring; 10 = minimal assistance and supervision; 15 = independent
9. Motility	0 = immobile; 5 = wheelchair independent for > 45 m; 10 = walks with help of one person > 45 m; 15 = independent for > 45 m, may use an aid (e.g., walking stick) except frame
10. Stairs	0 = unable; 5 = needs help or supervision; 10 = independent, may use aid

This is a numerical scale containing 10 fields, with total points ranging from 0 (totally dependent) to 100 (totally independent). The instructions for using the Barthel index correctly are as follows:
- the index must be used to record what a patient can really do, NOT what he/she might be able to do;
- the main scope is to establish the level of independence from any aid, whether physical or verbal, however minimal and for whatever reason;
- the need for supervision means that the patient is NOT independent;
- a patient's performance should be established using the best data available. The usual sources are direct questioning of the patient, his or her friends and relatives and nurses, but direct observation and common sense are also important. A direct examination is not necessary;
- performance in the previous 24-48 hours is usually important, but occasionally longer periods will also be relevant;
- unconscious patients should receive 0 for all items, even if they are not yet incontinent;
- intermediate categories mean that the patient participates with more than 50% of his or her energy;
- use of aids to be independent is allowed.

Nevertheless, a fairly recent study [25] in The Netherlands shows that non-survivors of intensive care (293 out of 2,578 patients in the study) mainly die because vital (artificial) support is withheld or withdrawn, and that this often occurs without essential information, due to a lack of documentation or inconsistencies with it, particularly in terms of the patient's wishes, and often without his or her family's involvement.

The search for statistical and numerical outcome markers is always a difficult task when the markers are to be used to choose between life and death for a particular individual. But the constant futility and frustration that accompany the care we provide to very ill patients is part of the daily routine for each and every one of us.

Just as we give extra importance to any gain in life that a potentially costly drug (such as activated protein C) may have demonstrated in the most relevant clinical studies, we give just as much importance to numbers and statistics that are able to predict the success of intensive care for patients in the advanced stages of functional degeneration. If accurate markers exist, or if they soon will, the way in which we provide intensive care will have to take this into account in order to draw a clear line between care and persistence.

If there is an upper limit to the relationship between resources and consumption within healthcare and social systems, and if all social systems – from the most advanced to those with the least resources – must in some way consider the end use of such resources, then the concept of triage will be viewed as it is on the battlefield, in theatres of war, in disasters and in situations involving multiple victims. In such cases the choices made are sometimes astonishing, but they are based on the idea that those with greater chances of survival should be first in line for treatment, following criteria that are standardised and recognisable and therefore ethical.

1.6 End of Life

It is unsurprising to include this type of reflexion in conclusion to such a complex and delicate subject.

The role of intensive care specialists is often central in deciding upon the level of care to be given to a particular patient, and often in deciding whether treatment is appropriate if the patient is too healthy or too ill to reasonably expect intensive care.

This is beyond the realm of a traditional and easily understandable approach to illness: diagnosis, treatment and stabilisation or recovery. Intensive care experts must contemplate the possibility of death – obviously the least painful form of death – in a cultural contest involving materialism, machinery, technology and, importantly, scotomisation as a patient's life draws to a close.

Faced as we are with advanced, chronic, degenerative diseases or terminal organ and system failure, we would like to respond to this difficult task with a quote from the SIAARTI guidelines (2006):

"(…) the caregiver is no longer in the presence of an ill person – a concept that fully embraces the real possibility of prolonging that person's life in a way that he or she finds acceptable – but in the presence of a dying person, a human being who is inevitably approaching the end of his or her life, whose needs must still be tended to and whose suffering must still be alleviated, ensuring dignity till the end, both in life and in death".

Bibliography

1. Carson SS (2003) The epidemiology of critical illness in the elderly. Crit Care Clin 19:605-617
2. Levin PD et al (2001) The process of intensive care triage. Int Care Med 27:1441-1445
3. Garrouste Orgeas et al (2006) Decision making process, outcome and 1 year quality of life of octogenarians referred for intensive care unit admission. Int Care Med 32:1045-1051
4. Martin GS et al (2006) The effect of age on the development and outcome of adult sepsis. Crit Care Med 34:15-21
5. Kass JE et al (1992) Intensive care unit outcome in the very elderly. Crit Care Med 20:1666-1671
6. Boumendil A et al. (2005) Treatment intensity and outcome of patients aged 80 and older in intensive care units: a multicenter matched-cohort study. J Am Geriatr Soc 53:88-93
7. Boumendil A et al (2004) Prognosis of patients aged 80 years and over admitted to medical intensive care unit Intensive. Care Med 30:647-654
8. Cohen I et al (1995) Investigating the impact of age on outcome of mechanical ventilation using a population of 41848 patient from a state-wide database. Chest 107: 1673-1680
9. Metnitz PG et al (2003) Critically ill patients readmitted to intensive care units – lessons to learn. Intensive Care Med 29:241-248
10. Hamel MB et al (1999) Patient age and decision to withhold life sustaining treatments from seriously ill, hospitalized adults. SUPPORT Investigators. Ann Intern Med 130:116-125
11. de Jonge E et al (2003) Intensive care medicine in the Netherlands 1997-2001. 1. Patient population and treatment outcome. Ned Tijdschr Geneeskd 147:1013-1017
12. Bo M et al (2003) Predictive factors of in-hospital mortality in older patients admitted in a medical intensive care unit. J Am Geriatr Soc 51:529-533
13. Jacobs DG (2003) Practice management guidelines for geriatric trauma: the EAST practice management guidelines. J Trauma 54:391-416
14. de Rooij SE et al (2006) Short term and long term mortality in very elderly patients admitted to an intensive care unit. Intensive Care Med 32:1039-1044
15. Torres OH et al (2006) Short and long term outcomes of older patients in intermediate care units. Intensive Care Med 32:1052-1059
16. Poses RM et al. (1996) Prediction of survival of critically ill patients by admission comorbidity. J Clin Epidemiol 49:743-747
17. Landi F (2000) Body mass index and mortality among hospitalized patients. Arch Intern Med 160:2641-2644
18. Ely EW (2003) Optimizing outcomes for older patients treated in the intensive care unit. Intensive Care Med 29:2112-2115
19. Bo M, Massaia M, Raspo S et al (2003) Predictive factors of in-hospital mortality in older patients admitted to a medical intensive care unit. J Am Geriatr Soc 51:529-533.
20. Mayer Oakes SA et al (1991) Predictors of mortality in older patients following medical intensive care: the importance of functional status. J Am Geriatr Soc 39:862-866
21. Somme D et al (2003) Critically ill old and the oldest old patients in intensive care: short and long term outcomes. Intensive Care Med 29: 2137-2143
22. Ehlenbach WJ (2010) Association between acute care and critical illness hospitalization and cognitive function in older adults. JAMA 303:763-770
23. Hennessy D et al (2005) Outcomes of elderly survivors of intensive care: a review of the . literature. Chest 127:1764-1774
24. Frick S et al. (2003) Medical futility: predicting outcome of intensive care unit patients by nurses and doctors: a prospective comparative study. Crit Care Med 31:456-461
25. Spronk P et al (2009) The practice of and documentation on withholding and withdrawing life support: a retrospective study in two Dutch intensive care units. Critical Care and trauma 109: 841-846

Is It Still Worth Treating At-Risk Patients with Perioperative Goal-Directed Haemodynamic Therapy?

2

Biagio Allaria

2.1 Introduction

The principle behind the belief that Goal-Directed Haemodynamic Therapy (GDHT) is the key to reducing mortality rates, complications and length of stay (LOS) in at-risk patients undergoing surgery (mainly abdominal, chest or vascular surgery for multiple trauma, sepsis and, generally speaking, surgery in which significant blood loss is expected) is that surgical stress can be overcome only with an oxygen delivery index (DO_2I) that is adjusted for metabolic requirements ($CaO_2 \cdot CI \cdot 10 = \geq 600$ mL/m^2/min). Oxygen supply to tissues may otherwise be insufficient, particularly in certain parts of the body (especially the intestines), and may lead to complications (e.g. chronic paralytic ileus) that in turn trigger other disorders (e.g. tachycardia, hypotension, myocardial ischemia) which at the very least prolong LOS but may even increase mortality rates.

This premise is strongly supported by observations made a while ago by Shoemaker et al. [18], which showed how high-risk patients who survive surgery have elevated Cl (4.5 L/min/m^2), DO_2I (> 600 mL/min/m^2) and VO_2I (> 170 mL/min/m^2). Shoemaker clearly demonstrated how these parameters are of much greater importance than those commonly used as a guide for treatment in these patients, namely arterial blood pressure, central venous pressure (CVP) and hourly diuresis. These observations influence the decision to use DO_2I as the primary treatment guide in seeking to obtain DO_2I values of 600 mL/m^2/min in any possible way (infusion and, in some cases, amines).

Some years later Boyd et al. [1] also made a similar declaration. In their study they observed two groups of patients: the first was treated with infusions

B. Allaria (✉)
Past Director of Critical Care Department
Istituto Nazionale per lo Studio e la Cura dei Tumori - National Cancer Institute, Milan, Italy
e-mail: biagio.allaria@tiscali.it

Biagio Allaria (ed.), *Practical Issues in Anesthesia and Intensive Care*
© Springer-Verlag Italia 2012

and possibly dopexamine to achieve and maintain DO_2I levels of approximately 600 mL/min/m², whereas the second group received conventional treatment and monitoring. DO_2 was controlled by means of a Swan-Ganz catheter. The objectives of the study were to reduce the mortality rate at 28 days as well as the number of complications. Both were reduced in the group receiving GDHT, but of particular interest was the fall in mortality from 22.2% to 5.7%. The patients treated by Boyd were on the whole serious cases, as demonstrated by the fact that the mortality rate was higher in the control group. This is very important as it shows how an obviously complicated control strategy, from an organisational perspective, was implemented in these patients and yielded important results.

2.2   How to Prevent Pulmonary Oedema Due to GDHT. Are Amines Actually Useful?

As will be discussed below, there are many ways to monitor DO_2I, including non-invasive methods, but the added value of using Swan-Ganz catheters is that they enable monitoring of pulmonary capillary pressure (PCP). This is perhaps a more useful parameter for avoiding overloading which can be a genuine risk when GDHT is implemented. It is not easy to decide when to abandon the infusion strategy and switch to an inotropic strategy if the desired DO_2I level has not yet been reached.

The study by Wilson et al. [24] sheds some light on the matter. Although it involved only a small number of patients, it is interesting because, in order to maintain DO_2I levels of 600 mL/min/m², the authors included another parameter called wedge pressure (WP), which they sought to maintain below 12 mmHg. But since the single most useful parameter is not WP by PCP, which is a few mmHg higher than WP, we can surmise that in the study by Wilson et al., PCP was maintained below 16-17 mmHg. The objective of this strategy is clear: to maintain PCP levels that prevent overloading as much as possible. Therefore, in this study infusions were administered until the critical DO_2I level was reached, but if it was not reached, inotropic treatment was added (dopexamine in one group of patients, adrenaline in another). The mortality rate was 17% in the control group, 4% in those receiving GDHT plus dopexamine, and 2% in those receiving GDHT plus adrenaline. These results are certainly extraordinary.

More clarification is needed. It may be inaccurate to switch from infusions to inotropic agents based on the numerical data for WP at 12 mmHg. WP is influenced not only by the preload but also by compliance of the left ventricle. Left ventricular hypertrophy with low compliance can raise WP levels to above 12 mmHg even when the preload is inadequate.

Some studies [13] have used this principle to give bolus administrations of plasma volume expanders and to continue with infusions although the heart does not respond to the fluid challenge with an increase in stroke volume (SV). This behaviour is significant for a heart that is on the ascending part of the

Frank Starling curve and which therefore improves its supply by increasing the preload.

We stated above that the decision to maintain elevated DO_2I levels in perioperative phases for at-risk patients arises from the observation that those who survive in such cases have higher DO_2I levels. But why is this so? It is based on the fact that VO_2 in perioperative phases ranges from 110 mL/m² at rest before surgery to 170 mL/m² after surgery, which amounts to the maintenance of an extended effort [15]. This type of VO_2 is maintained by an increase in Cl and O_2ER (oxygen extraction ratio). If metabolic requirements are higher than the possible increase in CI or O_2ER, the entire compensation relies on the preloading of anaerobic mechanisms of energy supply with a resulting ease in the onset of tissue hypoxia. However, patients in whom flow cannot be adjusted according to metabolic requirements in perioperative phases experience more complications and a higher mortality rate, as Shoemaker et al. [18] already demonstrated more than twenty years ago.

In most of the cases we came across, the administration of fluids allows DO_2I to rise even if the critical level of 600 mL/m²/min is not always reached. This is because blood loss and vasodilation from anaesthesia lead to a disproportion relationship between the circulatory bed and the mass contained on it, with a fall in venous return that is later reduced by mechanical ventilation with intermittent positive pressure. However, a number of different effects have been observed in certain patients, particularly those with known chronic cardiac insufficiency or those in whom myocardial ischemia has been established in intra- or postoperative phases: infusions not only increase SV, but can even reduce it. In such cases, the use of inotropic agents can be decisive. However, if inotropic agents are used, it must be remembered that administration is not without risks. Dobutamine, for instance, often triggers tachycardia, which is another risk factor if higher peaks are reached [10].

However, a more recent study [11] has compared the results of optimising DO_2I using infusions alone with the results of optimisation using dobutamine too in patients with cardiac insufficiency. In subjects who only received infusion, DO_2I levels during surgery are clearly inadequate, with the lowest level (just over 400 mL/m²/min) observed six hours after surgery. Patients receiving infusions and dobutamine had intraoperative levels that were substantially higher than 600 mL/m²/min during surgery; the lowest levels were often also reached six hours after surgery, but these were around 500 mL/m²/min and a satisfactory DO_2I level was restored after seven or eight hours. Patients treated with infusions and dobutamine had fewer postoperative complications and better outcomes.

The value of combination treatment with infusions and inotropic agents (dobutamine or dopexamine) has sparked the question as to whether or not these inotropic agents have any advantages themselves, regardless of the DO_2I levels that can be reached with them. There are certainly reports in the literature that support an anti-inflammatory effect for these amines and a protective action on microcirculation and splanchnic circulation [4].

These hypotheses do not seem to be fully backed up in the literature. For example, Stone et al. [22], in a study involving at-risk patients undergoing abdominal surgery and receiving haemodynamic control using the oesophageal Doppler technique, treated a group of patients with infusions alone and another with infusions and low doses of dopexamine. No difference was found between the two groups in terms of complications, LOS or outcome.

It is necessary to emphasise that the addition of an inotropic vasodilator such as dobutamine may cause undiagnosed hypovolemia and require later infusions, which are certainly useful and necessary in such cases. The effects of dobutamine, which are both harmful (hypotension) and useful (diagnosis of latent hypovolemia with the possibility of correction), may clarify some of the advantages of using it, irrespective of the anti-inflammatory effect, the protective effect on microcirculation or the exacerbating effect on DO_2I.

So far we have spoken of the need to adjust DO_2I according to the body's metabolic requirements and of existing reports in the literature on the efficacy of this adjustment in terms of reducing complications and LOS and improving outcomes. We also highlighted the need to avoid overloading by "dynamically" controlling SV: it is infused as long as it increases, with no significant rise in CVP and/or WP.

However, in critical patients receiving mechanical ventilation (as in intraoperative phases and the first hours after surgery of "at-risk patients"), the increase in CI that we use as an indicator of the validity of filling can be the cause of pulmonary oedemas. There are therefore two more important disorders that occur in at-risk patients in perioperative phases: flow deficit, especially splanchnic and coronary, and pulmonary oedema with resulting iatrogenic overflow, especially if damage to the alveolar-capillary barrier occurs at the same time.

We are used to thinking of damage to the barrier in patients with acute respiratory distress syndrome (ARDS), but it also occurs in much more common situations. For example, it is known that atelectatic pulmonary effects occur just one hour after mechanical ventilation in general anaesthesia. Tissue hypoxia, which occurs in the atelectatic zones, recalls neutrophils from the general circulation that are dangerously activated by pulmonary macrophages and become harmful to the alveolar-capillary barrier. The resulting overflow leads to oedemas even when the response of SV to the fluid load seems to be positive. This concept applies chiefly to patients with sepsis, but can be extrapolated to all at-risk patients receiving mechanical ventilation.

The findings of two recently published studies are convincing in this respect. The first concerns the fluid regimen instituted in cases of sepsis [5]. It stresses that generous administration of fluids is vital in the initial phases of treatment, but recommends a restricted fluid regimen in later stages. The title of the work, "Fluid therapy in resuscitable sepsis: less is more!", is itself indicative of the authors' certainty. But since one of the most feared complications in the postoperative phase in at-risk patients, especially in some diseases (peritonitis due to colon perforation and acute pancreatitis, for example) is ARDS, it is extremely important to know if overflow can contribute to it.

From this perspective the work by Xiaoming et al. published in 2008 in *Chest* is particularly interesting, as it analyses the most important risk factors for ARDS in patients receiving mechanical ventilation [25]. The authors studied 789 patients without ARDS who received mechanical ventilation for a variety of reasons, and identified the causes that have been influential in causing ARDS as a subsequent complication. Therefore, in 177 patients with ARDS, the most important risk factor is a positive fluid balance.

With this in mind, it is clearly important to be aware of the factors that influence the formation of pulmonary oedemas. Few authors have reported that one of these factors is tachycardia. Normally, during systole, the hydrostatic pressure of the capillaries increases, overcoming oncotic pressure, and a small amount of water enters the interstitial tissue. During diastole, the opposite occurs and water re-enters the circulation. Since diastole is longer than systole, the pulmonary interstitial tissue remains fairly dry. But in patients with persistent tachycardia, diastole shortens, the re-entry of interstitial fluid into the circulation becomes more difficult, and oedemas are triggered. The clinical case described by Lee in his book *The Pulmonary Circulation* [9] is interesting in this respect. While inserting a cardiac catheter into a patient with aortic stenosis, he reported acute dyspnoea following emotional tachycardia. Lee is convinced that the duration of diastole is important in the onset of pulmonary oedema, and did not administer any diuretics, as each one of us would have done, but instead administered an intravenous bolus of propranolol. Tachycardia was resolved along with dyspnoea. This case does not definitely imply the indiscriminate use of beta blockers in patients with aortic stenosis and dyspnoea, but is an indication of the importance of the duration of diastole in causing oedema.

Another, and perhaps the most important, factor in causing oedema is hydrostatic pressure in capillary circulation, i.e. PCP. The tradition of considering pulmonary capillary occlusion pressure (PCOP), or WP, to be interchangeable with PCP is too widespread. In reality, PCP is a few mmHg higher than WP in certain situations, such as ARDS, and it is not uncommon to find a difference of 7-8 mmHg between them. This is not only theoretical. It is clear to anyone that if a WP of 15 mmHg can be considered acceptable even in patients in whom damage to the alveolar-capillary barrier is suspected, a real PCP of 22-23 mmHg that can potentially cause pulmonary oedema cannot be judged satisfactory.

2.3 What Are the Alternatives to the Swan-Ganz Catheter in Implementing GDHT?

Due to the importance of monitoring PCP as well as DO_2I during perioperative phases in at-risk patients, it is clear that the only way to monitor both is with a Swan-Ganz catheter (pulmonary artery catheter, PAC). This type of monitoring, however, involves a series of problems that cannot be downplayed.

Firstly, the catheter is often inserted the day before surgery and kept in place at least 48 hours afterwards, including for the transfer of at-risk patients to ICUs for 3-4 days. The need for transfer to an ICU is influenced by two factors: (1) to protect the patient from possible complications of PAC, especially arrhythmias caused by dislocation of the catheter; (2) to take advantage of the opportunities to monitor the patient that are possible only with correct management of the monitoring techniques, which can only be done by specialists. Secondly, according to some works in the literature, there is a growing belief that PAC does not offer advantages in the management of critical patients. In reality this is refuted by the positive results obtained for the Swan-Ganz catheter in GDHT.

It therefore seems that the use of a Swan-Ganz catheter by specialists and with clear objectives, the existing control system is much more complete today. However, because of the difficulties related to the need to fill ICUs with this type of patient, the possibility of obtaining acceptable results without using Swan-Ganz catheters is increasing, mainly by means of the cardiac index (CI) and resulting DO_2I levels, which can be obtained non-invasively, as we shall see, with data from CVC and by limiting monitoring to the intraoperative period.

With this type of monitoring it is possible to explore the suitability of O_2 delivery for the body's needs, whether by estimating the amount of DO_2I by seeking to bring it towards the 600 mL/m²/min limit, or by monitoring $SCvO_2$ (SO_2 in the superior vena cava) which is closely correlated to SVO_2 and therefore provides us with the means by which the body can possibly use the mechanism of extraction of O_2 to attempt to maintain sufficient oxygenation. This type of monitoring, however, does not enable hydrostatic pressure to be estimated in the pulmonary capillary circulation and therefore does not alert us when dangerous limits for the onset of oedema are exceeded.

The alternatives to Swan-Ganz, which are currently used more often in at-risk surgery patients for haemodynamic optimisation, cannot be described as non-invasive but rather as "minimally invasive". The first alternative involves three monitoring systems based on analyses of the arterial pulse profile: LiDCO, PRAM and Vigileo. The first requires a control measurement with a lithium dilution that is used as a reference and must be repeated every eight hours; the second and third do not require any reference measurements and provide beat-to-beat SV data only when a cannula is inserted into the radial artery.

The second method is based on transpulmonary thermodilution (PiCCO), requires a CVC and, in general, insertion of a cannula into the femoral artery. It was one of the first monitoring systems to be implemented internationally as an alternative to the Swan-Ganz catheter and has the advantage of providing, in addition to flow data (SV, CI), extremely useful volumetric data for assessment of the preload (global end diastolic volume, GEDV, intrathoracic blood volume, ITBV). It is also particularly useful in implementing GDHT.

The third method is based on measuring flow in the descending aorta via a Doppler catheter inserted into the oesophagus. Two instruments are available: CardioQ, which measures aortic flow velocity using the Doppler catheter and calculates SV by manually inputting data (sex and age) with which the instrument calculates the diameter of the aorta; the second (HemoSonic) measures the diameter of the aorta via ultrasound and, with the Doppler catheter, measures the flow velocity, thereby directly obtaining the value of beat-to-beat SV. Since both systems estimate only the part of SV that passes through the descending aorta, ignoring the percentage that is directed to the supra-aortic trunks, it is more accurate to define these methods as measurements the flow of the descending aorta. Since, however, it is known that approximately 25%-30% of the capacity is distributed to the supra-aortic trunks, to obtain the entire capacity it is necessary to add the missing 25-30%, which the instruments do automatically.

Theoretically the HemoSonic system is more accurate, since it can directly measure the diameter of the aorta and its variations during the cardiac cycle, but it must be the case that if the measurement is not done correctly (which is possible despite assistance from the instruments), gross errors that are even greater than those caused by indirect measurement of the diameter by CardioQ cannot always be ruled out.

It therefore seems possible to say that the HemoSonic system is technologically more sophisticated and potentially more accurate; the CardioQ system is easier to use even by non-specialists. Both these methods have important limits for GDHT: planning for the need for an oesophageal catheter is difficult in preoperative estimates of DO_2I and in the postoperative phase of alert patients.

There are, nevertheless, also cases in the literature that support GDHT with an oesophageal Doppler technique in the intraoperative phase. For example, in at-risk patients undergoing orthopaedic surgery, the use of oesophageal Doppler has led to a reduction in LOS [20, 23]. Also in at-risk patients undergoing abdominal surgery, the use of oesophageal Doppler in intraoperative phases has enabled useful haemodynamic optimization with a consequent reduction in LOS and a faster return to solid foods [6, 3].

It must be added that, together with the DO_2I data to which we have repeatedly referred, other data are available for anaesthesia, such as oxygenation of venous blood in the superior vena cava ($SCvO_2$) and periodic lactate assays. These data appear to show that it is not imperative to reach supranormal DO_2I levels but not to achieve levels that trigger a reduction in $SCvO_2$ and do not increase lactate concentrations.

The work by Lobo et al. [12] is very interesting in this respect. The authors have used the LiDCO system for two groups of at-risk patients undergoing major general surgery. In the first group an attempt was made to reach a critical DO_2I of 600 mL/m²/min with the traditional method; in the second, a restricted fluid strategy was implemented, which was limited to compensating losses and maintaining a sufficient DO_2I with the help of dobutamine in order not to cause a fall in $SCvO_2$ and/or a rise in lactate.

Even with low intraoperative DO_2I levels, patients with a restricted fluid strategy had postoperative DO_2I levels that were very similar to those of patients receiving the supranormal DO_2I strategy and could boast a decidedly lower proportion of complications (2% versus 20%). These results raise the question we already highlighted of whether overflow related to GDHT can itself reduce the advantages.

The work by Lobo et al. [12] is a good combination of the need to adjust DO_2I according to metabolic requirements and a fluid restriction strategy that protects patients from complications resulting from oedemas and, in particular, introduces a concept that we have always believed, namely that all patients, especially those at risk, must be individually monitored with multi-parameter analyses that include DO_2I as well as $SCvO_2$ (in the absence of SVO_2), lactate, the ST segment on the ECG, oesophageal temperature, $ETCO_2$, blood pressure and heart rate, in order that all these parameters (to which we can add routine controls of urinary sodium in patients with confirmed or suspected hypovolemia) remain within the limits of normal.

Achieving supranormal DO_2I levels is a short-cut to obtaining normal levels for the above parameters without necessarily controlling all of them, the advantages of which have been described in the literature. The disadvantages linked to overflow, however, are difficult to control without a Swan-Ganz catheter that enables PCP to be measured.

We cannot close this brief review of non-invasive measures without mentioning two non-invasive monitoring methods. Despite widespread use in other medicinal sectors, there are currently seldom used in perioperative phases. They are volumetric capnography and impedance cardiography.

Volumetric capnography uses rebreathing to measure the components of cardiac output that are involved in respiratory exchanges and which are equivalent to PCP (pulmonary capillary blood flow, PCBF). Using FiO_2 and SpO_2 estimated by means of a diagram, the shunt fraction (the amount of cardiac output not involved in the exchange) is added to PCBF to calculate the value of cardiac output. It is a very reliable method and has the advantage of measuring not only PCBF but also dead space (VD/VT), making it particularly useful in optimising mechanical ventilation. As with the oesophageal Doppler technique, evaluations cannot be made outside of the intraoperative phase, and patients are required to be intubated and receive mechanical ventilation. Even as an instrument known primarily as a guide for mechanical ventilation, since it allow continuous measurement of cardiac output and therefore DO_2I, it can be proposed for GDHT despite the restrictions in intraoperative phases. The CO_2 partial breathing method is conceptually subject to possible errors, and the optimum rebreathing time (which must be shorter with a high supply than with a low supply) is still under discussion [26], and it is known to be particularly accurate with a PCBG of between 3 and 6 L/min. By underestimating the supply above this range and administering below it [7], we observed that it can be used for the most common applications of general anaesthesia, bearing in mind that the literature is at variance.

Impedance cardiography is the only entirely non-invasive haemodynamic monitoring method that can be used in all perioperative phases. The impedance cardiography measurements are, in fact, registered using self-adhesive sensors (two on the neck and two on the lower chest) with no discomfort for the patient. The system can very easily be set up within a few minutes by a few members of staff. It is based on variations in impedance caused by the flow of blood through the aorta during each systole. A series of algorithms that have been improved over time enables the measurement of cardiac revolution times (pre-ejection time, ejection time, diastole time distinguishing isometric relapsation time from isotonic relapsation time), cardiac output and (manually inserting pressure values for HB and SpO_2) the parameters for these dependents (DO_2, SVR, LVSW). This measure is therefore conceptually adjusted for GDHT, even if it is necessary to remember that whereas sufficient data are now available in the literature to consider it valid in critical patients and particularly in the routine assessment of patients with chronic cardiac insufficiency, there are no sufficiently comprehensive studies on its use in general anaesthesia [22, 17, 19].

We shall not go into detail about the methods for guiding the refilling of the circulation in patients receiving mechanical ventilation with systolic pressure variation (SPV), stroke volume variation (SVV) or pulse pressure variation (PPV). These parameters are certainly useful as an infusion guide but do not enable conventional GDHT, which is generally not proposed on its own as a means of refilling but as a basis for reaching optimum DO_2I levels.

2.4   Which Patients Are "at Risk" in GDHT?

From the above it is clear that GDHT is a challenging approach. If it is applied as proposed initially, in order to increase DO_2I levels to above 600 mL/m²/min whether in preoperative or intraoperative or postoperative phases, it inevitably requires patients to be transferred to an ICU the day before surgery and to remain there for at least two days afterwards. This is a problem in many parts of the world, where there are not enough intensive care beds and, general speaking, no subintensive beds.

Even when simplified, haemodynamic monitoring during the intraoperative period alone, which, as we already mentioned, can be useful, is very similar and therefore at least some patients receiving treatment are not able to achieve stable DO_2I levels and require at least 24 hours of postoperative monitoring.

Therefore, considering the organisational difficulties of GDHT, the criteria by which patients are selected is fundamental.

A meta-analysis conducted a few years ago using 21 studies addressing haemodynamic optimisation in at-risk patients concluded that those who will gain clear advantages from GDHT have postoperative mortality rates of 20% or more and therefore are considered extremely critical cases [8]. However, while it is relatively easy to identify categories of patients in a meta-analysis, it is much more difficult to do so in the case of a single patient. In clinical practice there is a tendency to underestimate the risk faced because, after all, death immediately after surgery is quite rare and the complications that emerge in later phases are often not even known by anaesthetists and therefore, as we have said, tend to be underestimated.

A British study has demonstrated that high-risk patients make up only 12.5% of surgical procedures but it is in this minority of surgical patients that 80% of deaths occur [16]. What is particularly important in this study is that only 15% of these high-risk and high-mortality patients were admitted to intensive care. Perhaps this is why mortality rates were so high.

What is clear is that major abdominal surgery, chest surgery, vascular surgery, major orthopaedic surgery and traumatology, not to mention heart surgery particularly in elderly patients or those with diabetes, heart disease, vascular disease or sepsis, as well as haemorrhagic patients and those in whom large blood loss is expected, are considered at risk. In all these patients it is often difficult for DO_2I levels to be adjusted according to metabolic requirements, especially in postoperative phases when VO_2 increases suddenly and splanchnic and coronary hypoxia occur more easily.

For example, in major abdominal surgery, a considerable inflammatory reaction is almost always observed with a consequent increase in O_2 requirements to which the patient may not be able to respond. Some authors recommend a cardiopulmonary stress test to identify the possibilities available to the patient to overcome surgical stress by estimating the anaerobic threshold [15]. But even this diagnostic test cannot always be used in at-risk patients: it is particularly impractical in emergencies, and difficult to implement in outlying hospitals where this type of test is not routinely carried out; furthermore, in elective surgery and larger hospitals the time available to prepare patients is increasingly being reduced as the demand for rapid turnover rises.

We must therefore satisfy ourselves as far as possible by assessing patients' clinical and medical history, always remembering that there are perioperative phases in which discrepancies between DO_2I and metabolic requirements can become a matter of concern and are noticed and corrected promptly and with accuracy.

It was recently said of the increase in VO_2 that it occurs in postoperative phases of major abdominal surgery but practically every type of surgery is accompanied by this type of event. During anaesthesia there is a fall in VO_2 that allows the lowest theoretical relative DO_2I level to be tolerated, but after surgery VO_2 can rise considerably. For example, after minor orthopaedic surgery, a few minutes after suspension of allogeneic blood, VO_2 increases from 173 to 473 mL/min and, if shivering occurs on awakening, it further increases to 800 mL/min and spontaneous ventilation may reach 30 L/min [2].

Anyone can understand that these situations are critical for patients who are not spontaneously able to make the necessary adjustments according to metabolic requirements.

2.5   Conclusions

With our current knowledge we note that very high-risk patients (for example, cases of stercoraceous peritonitis with sepsis and known heart disease) must imperatively be monitored with Swan-Ganz catheters that alone enable not only monitoring of DO_2I and SVO_2 levels but also PCP. In patients with presumed damage to the alveolar-capillary barrier, only the Swan-Ganz catheter can enable optimisation of the flow, minimising the possibility of pulmonary oedema. For such patients the organisational burden of this type of monitoring is absolutely justified.

In patients in whom the critical nature is not real but potential (for example, a diabetic patient with known cardiac insufficiency requiring hip replacement surgery), the organisational effort for traditional GDHT is probably not suited, at least in quite a large number of hospitals that do not have enough ICU beds on subintensive monitoring areas. In such cases, limited GDHT during the intraoperative phase is entirely advisable. We have seen that even simplified GDHT has its advantages, especially by reducing the rate of complications and therefore of LOS.

Obviously even simplified GDHT requires control instruments that enable continuous measurement of cardiac output and therefore DO_2I, which is the basis of GDHT. These data, together with frequent controls of O_2 saturation in the superior vena cava ($SCvO_2$) and lactate assays, enable satisfactory haemo-dynamic balance conditions to be reached at the end of surgery, whether achieved with infusions alone or with additional amine administration.

We have seen that technology offers many possibilities to implement this type of monitoring. We would like to add that the cost-effective use of such technology is can be managed by any hospital or, at least by those with enough awareness to understand the magnitude of the problem.

Bibliography

1. Boyd O et al (1993) A randomized clinical trial of the effect of deliberate perioperative increase of oxygen delivery on mortality in high risk surgical patients. JAMA 270:2699-2707
2. Ciofolo MJ (1989) Changes in ventilation, oxygen uptake and CO2 out up during recovery from anesthesia. Anesthesiology 70:737-741
3. Conway DH et al (2002) Randomized controlled trial investigating the influence of intravenous fluid filtration using oesophageal Doppler monitoring during bowel surgery. Anaesthesia 57:845-849
4. De Baker D et al (2006) The effects of dobutamine on microcirculatory alterations in patients with septic shock are independent of its systemic effects. Crit Care 34:403-408.
5. Durairaj L et al (2008) Fluid therapy in resuscitated sepsis. Chest 133:252-263. Eur J Anaesth 24:1028-1033
6. Gan TJ et al (2002) Goal directed intraoperative fluid administration reduces length of hospital stay after major surgery. Anesthesiology 97:820-826
7. Gueret G et al (2007) Comparison of cardiac output measurements between NICO and the

pulmonary artery catheter during repeat surgery for total hip replacement. Eur J Anestesial 24:1028-1033

8. Kern JW et al (2002) Meta analysis of hemodynamic optimization in high-risk patients. Crit Care Med 30:1686-1692
9. Lee GDJ (1994) The pulmonary circulation. In: Wagner WW, Weir EK, The pulmonary circulation and gas exchange, Futura, New York
10. Lobo SM et al (2000) Effects of maximizing oxygen delivery on morbidity and mortality in high risk surgical patients. Crit Care Med 28:3396-3404
11. Lobo SM et al (2006) Prospective, randomized trial comparing fluids and dobutamine optimization of oxygen delivery in high risk surgical patients. Crit Care 10:872
12. Lobo SM et al (2008) Early optimisation of oxygen delivery in high-risk surgical patients . In: Vincente JL (ed), Yearbook of intensive care and emergency medicine, Springer, New York
13. Mythen MG et al (1995) Perioperative plasma volume expansion reduces the incidence of gut mucosal hypoperfusion during cardiac surgery. Arch Surg 130:423-429
14. Older P et al (1993) Preoperative evaluation of cardiac failure and ischemia in elderly patients by cardiopulmonary exercise testing. Chest 104:701-704
15. Older P et al (1999) Cardiopulmonary exercise testing as a screening test for perioperative management of major surgery in the elderly. Chest 116:355-362
16. Pearse RM et al (2006) Identification and characterization of the high risk surgical population in the United Kingdom. Crit Care 10:R 81
17. Sageman WS et al (2002) Equivalence of bioimpedance and thermodilution in measuring cardiac index after cardiac surgery. JCVA16:8-14
18. Shoemaker WC et al (1988) Prospective trial of supranormal values of survivors as therapeutic goals in high risk surgical patients. Chest 94:1176-1186
19. Silver MB et al (2004) Evaluation of impedance cardiography as an alternative to pulmonary artery catheterization in Critical ill patients. CHF 10(Suppl 2):17-21
20. Sinclair S et al (1997) Intraoperative intravascular volume optimisation and length of stay after repair of proximal femoral fracture: Randomized trial. BMJ 315:909-912
21. Stone MD et al (2003) Effect of adding dopexamine to intraoperative volume expansion in patients undergoing major elective abdominal surgery. Br J Anaesth 91:619-629
22. Van De Water J et al (2003) Impedance Cardiography – The next vital sign technology? Chest 123:2028-2033
23. Venn R et al (2002) Randomized controlled trial to investigate influence of the fluid challenge on duration of hospital stay and perioperative morbidity in patients with hip fractures. Br J Anaesth 88:65-71
24. Wilson J et al (1999) Reducing a risk of major elective surgery: randomized controlled trial of preoperative optimisation of oxygen delivery. BMJ 318:1099-1103
25. Xiaoming J et al (2008) Risk factors for ARDS in patients receiving mechanical ventilation for >48 h. Chest 188:853-861
26. Yern SJ et al (2003) Sources of error in noninvasive PCBF measurements by partial rebreathing. Anesthesiology 98:881-887

Abdominal Compartment Syndrome and Fluid Replacement: a Dog That Bites Its Own Tail?

3

Massimo Girardis and Emanuela Biagioni

3.1 Introduction

It's 5:50 in the evening and the phone rings in the ICU. "Hi, Massimo, I was wondering if you had any beds free. Someone has been brought back to the operating room after undergoing surgery at the beginning of the week, because he had wound dehiscence on one of the sutures with a build-up of necrotic material and pus around the pancreas. I wanted to bring him to you as I'm having trouble maintaining correct pressure and have given anaesthesia. I've been told that since this morning he has had difficulty breathing and saturation is low. I have had to provide PEEP and 60% oxygen. He can urinate but before being transferred he took Lasix on the recommendation of his cardiologist because pulmonary oedema was suspected. But I don't think that's right. CVP is 6 and there are no X-rays. I still haven't understood what they want to do, but so far they have only washed him; I'm sending you the cultures taken in the ward that were sent for microscopic analysis...". The reality is that we have no free beds in intensive care, and so begins the customary "dance" that leads to unplanned discharge of the patient: selection of a lower-risk patient (*what indicators? SOFA score, destination and good sense*), bed availability in intended ward (*always difficult*), preparation of patient and documents, communication with patients and parents. Meanwhile the trainee doctor says: "Do you not think that this year we have had a few too many repeated surgical procedures? Why?" (*perhaps it's true, I'll think about it*). Immediately afterwards the nurse says, "Doctor, do we have to prepare anything in particular?".

This is an example of a real situation and the two good questions asked are the aspects we have chosen to discuss in this chapter. This is a common prob-

M. Girardis (✉)
Department of Anesthesia and Intensive Care
University Hospital of Modena, Modena, Italy
e-mail: massimo.girardis@unimore.it

lem, which is not only difficult but also, at least for us, partly unclear: what to do and what not to do when treating a patient with shock who also has intra-abdominal hypertension or factors that promote intra-abdominal hypertension?

3.2   Definitions of Intra-Abdominal Hypertension and the Problem at Hand

After years of uncertainty and doubts, recent literature has finally established some common ground: since 2006 there are agreed definitions for intra-abdominal hypertension (IAH), abdominal compartment syndrome (ACS), and for the most accurate methods for measuring intra-abdominal pressure (Table 3.1) [1].

Table 3.1 Definitions of intra-abdominal hypertension (IAH) and abdominal compartment syndrome (ACS) (Cheatham, 2006)

Definition 1	Intra-abdominal pressure (IAP) is the pressure at steady state concealed within the abdominal cavity
Definition 2	Intra-abdominal pressure (IAP) corresponds to mean arterial pressure (MAP) minus IAP (APP = MAP-IAP)
Definition 3	The renal filtration gradient (FG) is equal to MAP − 2 x IAP
Definition 4	IAP should be expressed in mmHg and measured at end-expiration in the complete supine position after ensuring that abdominal muscle contractions are absent and with the transducer zeroed at the level of the mid-axillary line
Definition 5	The reference standard for intermittent IAP measurement is via a vesical catheter with a maximum instillation volume of 25 mL of sterile isotonic saline
Definition 6	Normal IAP is approximately 5-7 mmHg in critically ill adults
Definition 7	IAH is defined by a sustained or repeated IAP value of at least 12 mmHg
Definition 8	IAH is graded as follows: • Grade I: IAP 12-15 mmHg; • Grade II: IAP 16-20 mmHg; • Grade III: IAP 21-25 mmHg; • Grade IV: IAP > 25 mmHg
Definition 9	Abdominal compartment syndrome (ACS) is defined as an IAP value of more than 20 mmHg (with or without APP < 60 mmHg) that is associated with new organ dysfunction
Definition 10	Primary ACS is a condition associated with injury or disease in the abdominopelvic region that frequently requires early surgical or or radiological intervention
Definition 11	Secondary ACS refers to conditions that do not originate from the abdominopelvic region
Definition 12	Recurrent ACS refers to the condition in which ACS redevelops following previous surgical or medical treatment of primary or secondary ACS

ACS, abdominal compartment syndrome; *APP*, abdominal perfusion pressure; *IAH*, intra-abdominal hypertension; *IAP*, intra-abdominal pressure; *MAP*, mean arterial pressure.

Moreover, numerous epidemiological and pathophysiological data are available that should enable quantification of the phenomenon and understanding of it, but when the studies are analysed, it is understood that precise definitions have become (and we believe still is) very difficult to make. This is probably useful when writing scientific works but extremely difficult in everyday practice. For this reason, instead of entering into detail about the scope of definitions or the most correct saline volume to insert into a vesical catheter to measure abdominal pressure (see Table 3.1), we prefer to discuss the causes of abdominal hypertension and the pathophysiological aspects.

The premise with which we shall begin is that there are very few cases of anaesthesia or resuscitation for patients with IAH or a risk of IAH in their professional lives, even if we do not count injured patients. How many are there? This depends on the type of patient treated [2]: the estimated incidence of septic shock is approximately 50% [3], in surgical patients it drops to 40% [4], in those with liver transplant to 30% [5] and with various types of trauma to between 10% and 50% [6]. Some years ago we studied patients admitted to our ICU after emergency surgery, observing that 63% had IAH and of these 12% had ACS [7]. Returning to our example, to answer the doubt expressed by the trainee doctor we checked the database, which showed that in our ICU in recent years repeated surgery had indeed increased, together with patient age and comorbidities. All these factors increase the risk of IAH or ACS for patients (Table 3.2). Are we alone in this respect? Sifting through the data from the GiViTi Margherita Project it appears that in Italy the mean age of patients admitted to intensive care as well as comorbidities and the type of surgery have not changed in the last three years (www.marionegri.giviti.it). Colleagues from other departments disagree, but numbers are numbers.

Table 3.2 Risk factors for development of IAH and ACS [16]

A. Decreased abdominal wall compliance
Patient with mechanical breathing and/or ventilator dyssynchrony
Use of PEEP or presence of auto-PEEP
Basal pulmonitis-pleuritis
Elevated BMI
Pneumoperitoneum
Abdominal surgery, particularly with "tight" abdominal wall sutures
Prone positioning or other non-supine positions
Abdominal wall bleeding or muscle fascia haematoma
Correction of major hernia, gastroschisis or omphalocele
Burns with abdominal eschars
B. Increased abdominal contents
Gastroparesis
Gastric distention

(cont. →)

Table 3.2 (*continued*)

Ileus
Volvolus
Colonic pseudo-obstruction
Intra-abdominal/retroperitoneal haematoma
Intra-abdominal/retroperitoneal tumour
Enteral feeding
Laparotomy with post-traumatic damage control
C. Increased abdominal fluids, air or blood
Ascites
Abdominal infections (pancreatitis, peritonitis, abscesses)
Haemoperitonitis
Pneumoperitoneum
Major trauma
Peritoneal dialysis
D. Increased capillary permeability and fluid resuscitation
pH < 7.2
Body temperature < 33°C
Coagulopathy (platelet count < 50 x 10^3, PTT x 2 , PT INR > 1.5)
Multiple transfusion with trauma > 10 U EC/24 h
Sepsis, severe sepsis and septic shock
Major fluid resuscitation (> 5 L of colloids or > 10 L of crystalloids/24 h with increased capillary permeability and positive fluid balance)
Major burns

3.3   The Pathophysiology and Rationale of Treatment Decisions

The abdomen can be considered a closed box with rigid walls (costal arc, vertebrae, pelvis) as well as elastic walls (diaphragm, abdominal walls), and the pressure inside this box depends on its contents (directly proportional) and the compliance of the walls (inversely proportional). Any increase in the content (for example, an increase in the volume of the intestines, the presence of ascites or blood) or reduction in the compliance of the walls (for example, burns, interstitial oedema or abdominal surgery wounds) leads to an increase in IAH. With the introduction of these simple physical concepts, the main focus below is to consider IAH as a disease in itself capable of causing changes in organ function, as is the case with haemorrhage, sepsis or cardiac decompensation. Independently of the primary etiology (see Table 3.2), IAH influences pulmonary, cardiovascular, intestinal and renal function. Two other simple but important aspects are that pathophysiological changes are even observed for small increases in abdominal pressure and that these changes increase exponentially with the rise in abdominal pressure

(Fig. 3.1) [8]. We shall examine what this means in practice, starting with the abdominal organs.

3.3.1   Intestines and Kidneys

As with the brain in patients with endocranial hypertension, IAH causes a reduction in abdominal perfusion pressure (APP) (see Table 3.1) with the possible development of hypoperfusion and hypoxia in the kidneys and intestines. It is well known that the first clinical sign of IAH/ACS is oliguria and the organ that experiences insufficiency first and to the greatest extent is the kidney. The pathophysiological reason for renal insufficiency during ACS is complex, but certainly the reduction in renal blood flow caused by the rise in pressure in the renal veins mediated by the increase in IAP plays a fundamental role [9]. But as is well known, the kidney is often a minor actor who dies first in our films and, fundamentally, we do not worry about it. To us it is more interesting to see what happens in the intestines after hypoperfusion/hypoxia during IAH/ACS. This phenomenon, which is associated with the primary cause of IAH, can lead to a protective inflammatory response in the tissues with an increase in interstitial oedema in the organ and therefore a later rise in IAH and a fall in PPA. This form of secondary injury caused by hypoperfusion appears to be responsible for more complex forms of IAH/ACS, so that the term "acute abdominal distress syndrome" has been suggested in analogy with acute respiratory distress syndrome (ARDS) in the lungs [10]. Patients that are most likely to develop acute abdominal distress syndrome are those with septic shock in whom bacterial endotoxins and inflammatory cytokines cause splanchnic hypoperfusion and an increase in endothelial permeability with subsequent development of intestinal oedema and therefore of IAH.

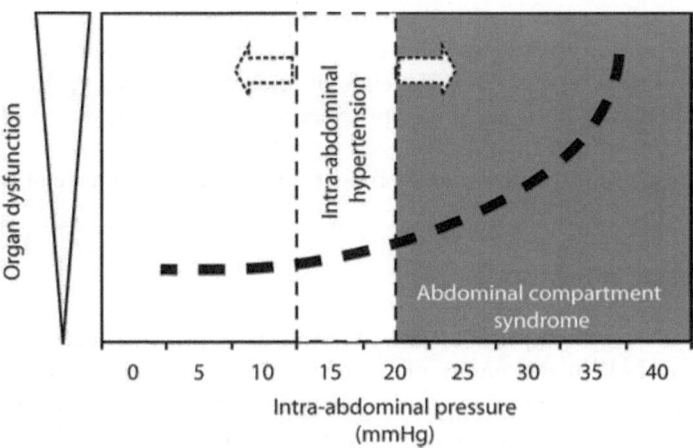

Fig. 3.1 Diagram showing the relation between intra-abdominal pressure and organ dysfunction

What are the repercussions of all this in clinical practice? The maintenance or improvement of APP are crucial objectives for the treatment of patients with IAH/ACS, in order to avoid later deterioration of IAH, the development of acute renal insufficiency and abdominal intestinal distress syndrome [11]. The problem that arises from this is to decide on the APP level that should be maintained or re-established. There are few studies that are available to clarify this point, and it should be remembered that there is a large amount of inter-individual variability that depends, obviously, on the patient's comorbidities. Despite this uncertainty, the currently recommended APP level for the maintenance of adequate organ perfusion ranges from 50 mmHg to 60 mmHg [12]. The solution may seem obvious enough: reduce IAP or increase MAP. Unfortunately the situation is not as simple as it looks (see also the paragraph on fluid treatment).

3.3.2 Respiratory System

Anyone who works in an operating room in intensive care on a daily basis knows very well that any increase in IAH leads to changes in respiratory function mediated by:
- cephalic movement of the diaphragm which causes a reduction in residual functional capacity;
- transmission of IAH to the intrathoracic region with an increase in pleural pressure;
- reduction in thoracic compliance due to a fall in abdominal compliance [13].

What does this mean in clinical practice for mechanical ventilation? It means that if the correct approach is not taken, i.e. by changing the ventilation strategy, these patients will develop hypoxia with a low ventilation/perfusion ratio. Therefore, especially in patients with ACS associated with ALI/ARDS, it must be remembered:
- to consider IAH when choosing PEEP (imposed PEEP = IAH);
- that pressure in the airways (Paw) detected at the patient's mouth is not transmural pressure (Ptm) that also depends on pleural pressure (Ppl) (for example, Ptm = Paw – Ppl), and that Ppl exacerbates the increase in IAP (approximately Ppl = IAP/2);
- to consider the use of muscle relaxants to reduce abdominal compliance [14].

3.3.3 Cardiovascular System

As with the respiratory system, it is clear enough in daily practice that every increase in transient IAP (for example, pneumoperitoneum) or persistent IAP (for example, ascites) causes cardiovascular changes that vary linearly with increased IAP. Increased intrathoracic pressure reduces venous return after an initial rise caused by compression of abdominal vessels and thus reduces cardiac output. Mean arterial pressure (MAP) is not a good indicator of perfusion in patients with IAH because, unlike what has already been said for PPA, compression of splanchnic vessels and the activation of the renin-angiotensin-aldosterone system can increase systemic vascular resistance with maintenance of normal MAP even with reduced cardiac output [15]. What should be done to avoid/treat these cardiovascular changes? The easiest answer, other than seeking if possible to reduce IAP, is to increase the circulating volume to raise venous return, but as we shall see later, this must be done carefully using accurate parameters and objectives. In fact, other than scant reliability of MAP as an indicator for organ perfusion, the increase of intrathoracic pressure means that cardiac preload parameters based on static measurements of pressure (CVP, PAOP) are largely unreliable and their use as absolute values for fluid replacement must be avoided because it can lead to inappropriate therapeutic decisions [16].

3.4   Medical Treatment of IAH/ACS: the Fluid Dilemma

The complete description of IAH/ACS goes beyond the scope of this text and readers should refer to the guidelines of the international conference on IAH/ACS (World Society of the Abdominal Compartment Syndrome - http://www.wsacs.org/). Figure 3.2, adapted from the original WSACS algorithm, summarises the medical treatment of IAH/ACS following a step-by-step logic for each of the treatment options. The rationale of any of these treatment choices is simple and has been covered in the previous paragraph. One of the more pressing problems remains to be discussed, and having heard anaesthetists and providers of resuscitation, it can have a great impact on the development/deterioration of IAH/ACS: how to resuscitate a patient with IAH/ACS and impaired organ perfusion (e.g. renal, splanchnic)? In essence, the last two sections of the therapeutic algorithm are shown in Figure 3.2. The problem arises because we have suggested two approaches, which are apparently contradictory:

- in patients with IAH/ACS it is vital to maintain adequate intravascular volume to avoid organ hypoperfusion caused by an increase in IAP (see above) that can later worsen the picture of IAH;
- aggressive fluid treatment and the maintenance of a positive balance are independent risk factors for the development of secondary IAH/ACS and for a rise in the likelihood of death [17, 18].

Therefore, it is necessary to find an "adequate" volume, not to be aggressive and avoid a positive balance. This is not at all easy. The solution, in our opinion, is to carefully monitor haemodynamic and organ perfusion parameters and to form resuscitation algorithms with precise objectives.

As already proposed for the cardiovascular system, the traditional static pressure parameters for preload and systemic pressure are little used in these patients. There are many alternatives, particularly to assess patients' capacity

IAH/ACS MEDICAL MANAGEMENT ALGORITHM

✓ The choice of medical treatment, listed below, is strongly related to the etiology of the patient's IAH/ACS and to the clinical situation. The appropriateness of each intervention should always be considered a priority in order to implement these interventions in various types of patients.
✓ The interventions should be applied in a stepwise fashion (from 1 to 4) until the patient's IAP decreases.
✓ If there is no response to medical treatment, you should continue to the next step

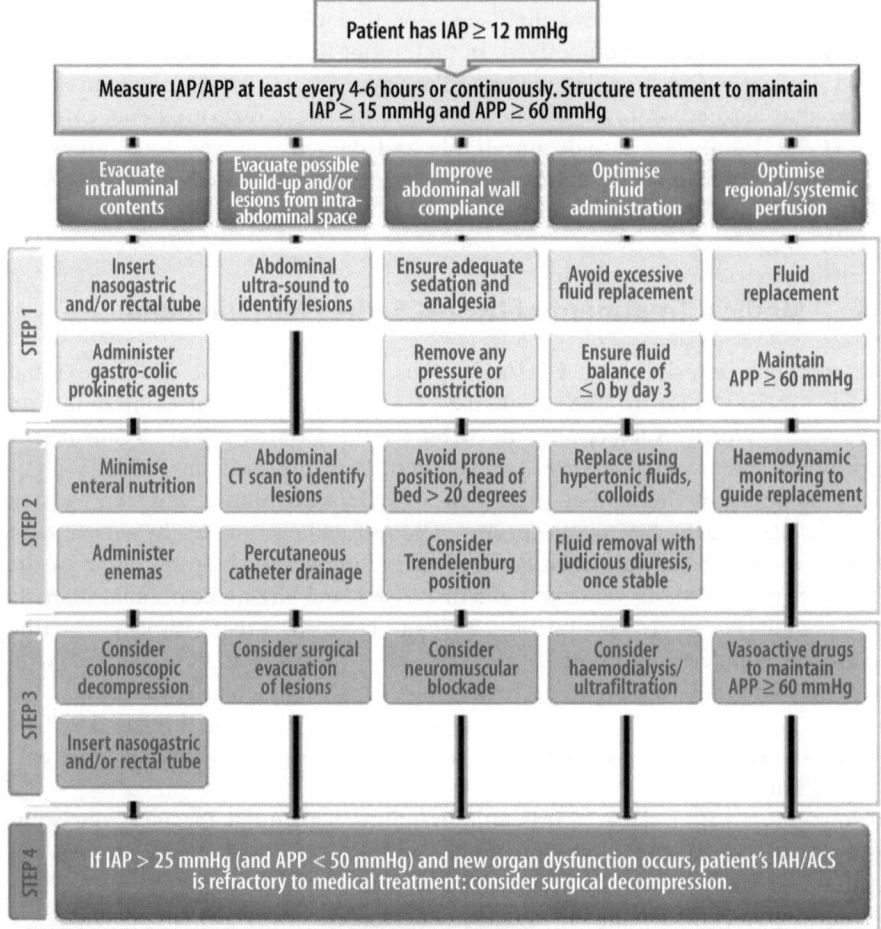

Fig. 3.2 Summary of protocol for medical treatment of IAH/ACS. From [6], amended

to respond to fluid treatment (e.g., the most correct form now used for pre-load): the measurement of cardiac volume (via echocardiogram and/or transpulmonary dilution) and dynamic parameters (e.g. variation in pulsatory pressure) have been shown to be reliable in the assessment of patients with IAH [19]. But it seems to us that these parameters are of little use, since in a patient in whom it is desired to avoid even a single millilitre of excess fluid, regular fluid treatment is required using parameters that assess cardiovascular function and organ perfusion function (e.g. cardiac output, haematic lactate, base excess, O_2 saturation in the mixed venous blood) [20]. If our patient showed no signs of hypoperfusion, on the other hand, it would have been of little use to know whether or not he responded to fluids because they were not administered. However, if the patient did have signs of hypoperfusion, the least amount of fluid possible would have been administered and vasoactive amines would have been used early on to guarantee adequate cardiac output and organ perfusion. It is necessary to clarify this approach, which is also recommended in international guidelines [6], but it has not yet been the subject of large-scale randomised prospective studies. As with small volume resuscitation for injured patients, however, this is based on sound pathophysiological principles.

Having defined the strategy for fluid administration, it will be seen that data are available for choosing the type of fluids. As expected, the use of synthetic or natural colloids and hypertonic crystalloids in patients with changes to endothelial permeability and IAH seems to have a protective effect compared to isotonic crystalloids, whether for the development/deterioration of IAH or for the likelihood of death [21, 22].

To summarise these concepts, we refer to the recommendations agreed by the conference [6] on the problem of fluid resuscitation:

- fluid resuscitation with hypertonic crystalloids and/or colloids must be considered in patients with IAH to prevent progression towards secondary ACS (1C);
- the volume of fluid resuscitation must carefully be monitored to avoid water overload (1B).

3.5 Conclusions

In this brief examination of the problems encountered by patients with IAH, we are able to answer the question asked by the nurse in reference to the case reported in the Introduction to this chapter: "Doctor, do we have to prepare anything in particular?". This is because we feel a little more prepared and can respond with what is needed:

- measure abdominal pressure immediately and then every 4-6 hours; if IAP > 12 mmHg, inform the doctor immediately;
- measure lactates and SvO2 every 4-6 hours and if there are signs of hypoperfusion monitor cardiac output (PiCCO or PAC);
- prepare synthetic colloids and if albuminaemia is low (< 2,0 mg/dL) request albumin;
- prepare a syringe pump for amine infusion;
- check water balance every 6 hours.

As a start this is not bad, but the nurse has already given us several dirty looks.

Bibliography

1. Malbrain ML, Cheatham ML, Kirkpatrick et al (2006) Results from the International Conference of experts on intra-abdominal hypertension and abdominal compartment syndrome. I. Definitions. Intensive Care Med 32:1722-1732
2. Malbrain ML, Chiumello D, Pelosi P et al (2004) Prevalence of intra-abdominal hypertension in critically ill patients: a multicentre epidemiological study. Intensive Care Med 30:822-829
3. Regueira T, Hasbun P, Rebolledo R et al (2007) Intra-abdominal hypertension in patients with septic shock. Am Surg. 73:865-70
4. Sugrue M, Jones F, Deane SA et al (1999) Intra-abdominal hypertension is an independent cause of postoperative renal impairment. Arch Surg 134:1082-1085
5. Biancofiore G, Bindi ML, Romanelli AM et al (2003) Postoperative intra-abdominal pressure and renal function after liver transplantation. Arch Surg 138:703-706
6. Cheatham ML, Malbrain ML, Kirkpatrick A et al (2007) Results from the International Conference of experts on intra-abdominal hypertension and abdominal compartment syndrome. II. Recommendations. Intensive Care Med 33:951-962
7. Busani S, Soccorsi MC, Poma C, Girardis M (2006) Intra-abdominal hypertension in nonelective surgery: a preliminary report. Transplant 38:836-837
8. Malbrain ML, Deeren D, De Potter TJ (2005) Intra-abdominal hypertension in the critically ill: it is time to pay attention. Curr Opin Crit Care 11:156-171
9. De Waele JJ, De Laet I (2007) Intra-abdominal hypertension and the effect on renal function. Acta Clin Belg Suppl:371-374
10. Kirkpatrick AW, Balogh Z, Ball CG et al (2006) The secondary abdominal compartment syndrome: iatrogenic or unavoidable? J Am Coll Surg 202:668-679
11. Cheatham ML, White MW, Sagraves SG et al (2000) Abdominal perfusion pressure: a superior parameter in the assessment of intra-abdominal hypertension. J Trauma 49:621-626
12. Malbrain ML. Abdominal perfusion pressure as a prognostic marker in intra-abdominal hypertension. In Vincent JL (ed) Yearbook of intensive care and emergency medicine. Springer-Verlag, Heidelberg, 2002, 792-414.
13. Ranieri VM, Brienza N, Santostasi S et al (1997) Impairment of lung and chest wall mechanics in patients with acute respiratory distress syndrome: role of abdominal distension. Am J Respir Crit Care Med 156:1082-1091
14. De Laet I, Hoste E, Verholen E, De Waele JJ (2007) The effect of neuromuscular blockers in patients with intra-abdominal hypertension. Intensive Care Med 33:1811-1814
15. Bloomfield GL, Blocher CR, Fakhry IF et al (1997) Elevated intra-abdominal pressure increases plasma renin activity and aldosterone levels. J Trauma 42:997-1004
16. De Laet LE, De Waele JJ, Malbrain ML (2009) How does intra-abdominal pressure afect the daily management of my patients. In: Vincent JL (ed) Yearbook of intensive care and emergency medicine, pp 629-645. Springer-Verlag, Heidelberg
17. McNelis J, Marini CP, Jurkiewicz A et al (2002) Predictive factors associated with the development of abdominal compartment syndrome in the surgical intensive care unit. Arch Surg 137:133-136
18. Balogh Z, McKinley BA, Cocanour CS et al (2003) Supranormal trauma resuscitation causes more cases of abdominal compartment syndrome. Arch Surg 138:637-642
19. Michard F, Alaya S, Zarka V et al (2003) Global end-diastolic volume as an indicator of cardiac preload in patients with septic shock. Chest 124:1900-1908
20. Gutierrez G, Wulf-Gutierrez ME, Reines HD (2004) Monitoring oxygen transport and tissue oxygenation. Curr Opin Anaesthesiol 17:107-117
21. Oda J, Ueyama M, Yamashita K et al (2006) Hypertonic lactated saline resuscitation reduces the risk of abdominal compartment syndrome in severely burned patients. J Trauma 60:64-71
22. O'Mara MS, Slater H, Goldfarb IW, Caushaj PF (2005) A prospective, randomized evaluation of intra-abdominal pressures with crystalloid and colloid resuscitation in burn patients. J Trauma 58:1011-1018

Acute Liver Failure in Intensive Care

4

Andrea De Gasperi, Patrizia Andreoni, Stefania Colombo, Paola Cozzi
and Ernestina Mazza

4.1 Definition, Epidemiology, Clinical Signs and Aetiology

Acute liver failure (ALF) is a rare syndrome characterized by sudden and acute hepatic injury which can be attributed to a number of different causes although not all of them are always clearly identifiable [1-13]. A severe compromise of parenchymal function is followed, at different intervals, by the onset of hepatic encephalopathy, serious haemostasis alteration and, in many cases, multiple organ failure. In the 70s the term FHF (*fulminant hepatic failure*) had been introduced to describe serious hepatic damage, in absence of known pre-existing hepatic disease, with subsequent onset of encephalopathy within 8 weeks. The syndrome was described as "potentially reversible" [1, 2, 12]. The definition proposed by O'Grady in 1993 and still used today recognizes that the onset of encephalopathy and of altered awareness at different degree is fundamental from a prognostic point of view [2, 12]. Elevated transaminase, hyperbilrubinemia, encephalopathy and serious coagulopathy are the main characteristics of ALF [1-7, 10]. All the identifying factors that have been proposed include the onset of encephalopathy in the course of ALF, the lack of pre-existing hepatic disease and the high incidence of spontaneous mortality (>85%). This pathology presents itself in a variety of ways and it may be a combination of different aetiologies, each producing a very different outcome. ALF is identifiable by a progressive bilirubin increase [1-7] within a time span of 7 days to 26 weeks after acute liver damage. Depending on the interval between the onset of jaundice and the clinical signs of encephalopathy, the syndrome is classified as hyper-acute (jaundice-encephalopathy interval: <7 days); acute (jaundice-encephalopathy interval: 8-28 days); sub-acute (jaundice-encephalopathy interval: 28 days-26

A. De Gasperi (✉)
2nd Anesthesia and Critical Care Service, Transplant Department
Ospedale Niguarda Ca' Granda, Milan, Italy
e-mail: andrea.degasperi@ospedaleniguarda.it

weeks). Bernal et al. [1] agree with this classification in the most recent review published on the subject.

Every year there are 2,000 new cases in the United States, 400 in the UK and an estimated 100 in Italy [1, 3, 11, 13]. Intensive treatment is well documented and must aim to identify, if possible, and/or remove, if possible, the leading cause of liver damage [4, 7, 10]. Artificial or bioartificial extracorporeal support, however conducted, should promote an improvement of the patient's condition, which in turn would promote hepatic regeneration and avoid organ and systemic complications [1, 4, 7, 10]. A liver transplant option should be considered for those patients with insufficient hepatic regeneration and such indication, in order to be effective, must be timely and appropriate (*vide infra*) [1, 9].

The syndrome's aetiology and different onset manifestations have significant implications with regard to both its clinical progression and outcome [1-14] (Table 4.1).

The onset of hepatic encephalopathy shows alterations of awareness and behaviour ranging from moderate confusion to deep coma without reflex [2, 12] (Table 4.2).

ALF is associated to alterations of haemodynamics (high cardiac output, low mean arterial pressure, low systemic resistance) [7], of coagulation [15-17], of renal function, of gas exchange and of metabolic profile (acidosis, hypoglycemia) [1, 6, 7, 10]. An increased tendency to infection has also been observed, bacterial and mycotic infections in particular; the onset of multiple organ failure syndrome takes in fact shape [1, 3-10].

The accumulation of inflammatory cytokines, of hydrosoluble toxins (ammonia and mercaptan) and of hydrophobic substances bound to albumin (bilirubin, aromatic amino acids, endogenous benzodiazepines, bile salts, short-chain fatty acids) has a significant role in the onset of hepatic encephalopathy and, potentially, of cerebral oedema. High levels of nitric oxide (NO) and cytokines are associated with renal damage and cardiocirculatory alterations. Finally, the presence of oxidants is cause for increased capillary permeability and immunological profile alteration [6].

Table 4.1 Classification and evolution of acute hepatic failure

	Hyper-acute	Acute	Sub-acute
Jaundice-encephalopathy interval	0-1 week	1-4 weeks	4-12 (up to 26) weeks
Coagulopathy extent	+++	++	+
Jaundice extent	+	++	+++
Intracranial hypertension	++	++	+/-
Survival without urgent OLT	Good (>60%)	Moderate (50%)	Low (10-20%)
Most frequent causes	Paracetamol, Hepatitis A and E	Hepatitis B	Liver damage, no paracetamol

Table 4.2 Stages of hepatic encephalopathy

	Description	Clinical signs	GCS
I	Neurasthenia	Fatigue syndrome, depression confusion, behaviour and mood alterations	15
II	Drowsiness	Flapping tremor, apraxia, asterixis, torpor, lethargy, confusion, uninhibited behaviour	11-13
III	Sopor	Reduced ability to answer, ability to follow only simple orders, uncoordinated speech, apraxia, asterixis, Babinski, possible loss of protective reflexes, altered EEG (triphasic waves)	8-13
IVa	Coma	Response only limited to painful stimuli, decerebration	3-8
IVb	Deep coma	No response to pain, low signal or isoelectric EEG	3

Since liver transplant became a recognized form of treatment there has been a great change in the natural progression of ALF [1-5, 9] (Fig. 4.1).

Liver transplant (OLT, *orthtopic liver transplantation*) can address multiple organ failure and associated systemic consequences and can therefore significantly modify ALF prognosis [1, 9]. Pre-OLT mortality ranged between 70 and 90%. Today, the average survival for the transplanted patient is close to 80% while 20-25% of patients experience spontaneous recovery [1-13]. It is also important to underline how an "optimal" intensive treatment, even without liver transplant, has brought the survival rate to over 60% for some forms of ALF namely those induced by hepatitis A, paracetamol, ischaemia or associated with pregnancy [1-11].

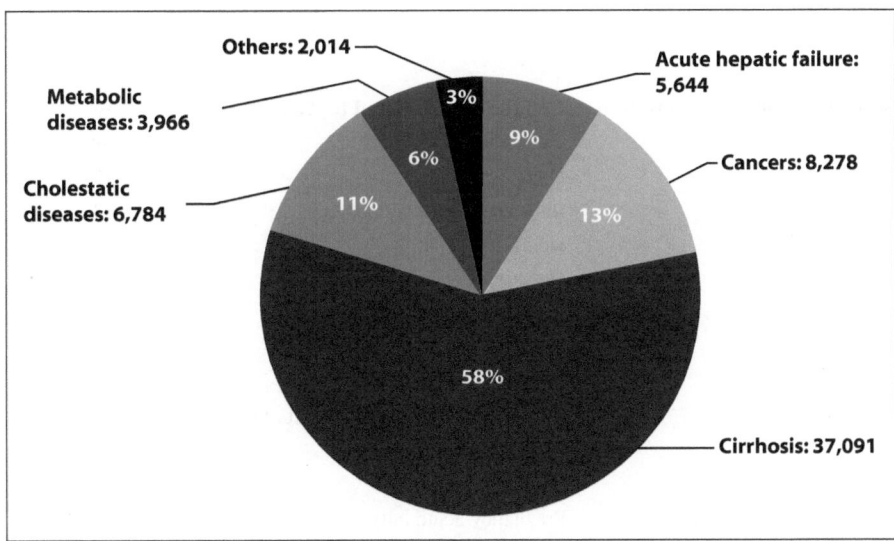

Fig. 4.1 Primary hepatic pathologies leading to liver transplant in Europe, January 1998-December 2007

ALF is caused by varied aetiology: viral, metabolic, auto-immune, toxic, vascular (Table 4.3) and it develops through direct cytotoxic or cytopathogenic damage [10]. Aetiology remains however unknown in a significant percentage of cases. Different noxae prevail in adults as opposed to paediatric patients and also in relation to geographical areas (Europe and North America not as Asia and South America). In Europe (particularly in UK) and in North America a significant number of cases is due to paracetamol ingestion and to other drugs' idiosyncratic effect. Paracetamol-induced ALF usually has hyper-acute onset, often with concurrent MOF. No criteria are contemplated in this case for urgent liver transplant (see King's College criteria) but given the fact that there is regenerative potential [1, 8] a prognosis based on medical treatment alone remains favourable. The prevalence of ALF caused by viral hepatitis varies depending on the period of time under consideration and on the geographic location. Hepatitis B prevails in Asia and Africa and it has abated (though still present) in Europe and North America; hepatitis A prevails in children in Asia and Africa. Hepatitis E has been placed amongst the causes of ALF for a few years. It has a low incidence (< 1%), it is frequently hyper-acute, it has been observed in older, run-down or immunosuppressed patients, mortality is usually not high but without urgent liver transplant it can be higher than 50% [1]. Extremely rare but documented forms of ALF are linked to C virus hepatitis [1].

Other conditions that could cause ALF are some metabolic disorders (Wilson's disease, Reye syndrome), thrombophilia conditions (Budd-Chiari syndrome), pregnancy microangiopathy (HELPP syndrome, acute fatty liver in pregnancy), some autoimmune disorders often diagnosed as such by exclusion [1]. Strawitz et al. [88] have very recently proposed a systematized autoimmune-ALF diagnosis by histological and clinical method; there are in fact forms that

Table 4.3 Causes of acute liver failure

Conditions associated to ALF	%
Paracetamol	39
Undetermined causes	17
Idiosyncratic reactions	13
Ischaemic hepatitis	6
Hepatitis B	7
Hepatitis A	4
Autoimmune hepatitis	4
Wilson's disease	3
Mushroom poisoning (Amanita Phalloides)	2
Budd-Chiari syndrome	2
HELPP syndrome	1
Pregnancy acute fatty liver	1
Metastatic disease	1
Other (incl. haemophagocytic syndrome)	2

are classified as autoimmune by exclusion of evident causes, when seronegativity is present and when there is no documented toxicology. An extremely rare form is linked to haemophagocytic syndrome. Viral forms linked to the herpes virus (simplex; zoster; varicella), parvovirus B19, cytomegalovirus (CMV) or Epstein-Barr virus (EBV) are quite rare but have been recorded [1].

The direct cytotoxic effect on hepatocytes is linked to virus A hepatitis, to drugs (paracetamol, nimesulide, flutamide, cyproterone), to toxins as in the case of mushrooms poisoning, to carbon tetrachloride and to illegal euphorising substances found in young people's environments (recreational drugs such as 3,4-methylenedioxymethamphetamine better knows as ecstasy, a synthetic amphetamine) [14]. Reference is made to cytopathic effect when hepatocyte necrosis is immune-mediated (e.g. hepatitis B-induced necrosis).

4.2   Prognosis, Indications for Transferral to Intensive Care and for Transplant, Treatment

As already mentioned, prognosis varies depending on aetiology and age. It is more favourable in the under 65 in case of ALF linked to hepatitis A or E, to paracetamol or appearing during pregnancy; it is severe (above 70% mortality) in case of idiosyncratic syndrome or if hepatitis B-induced. The degree of encephalopathy is a most relevant factor in predicting outcome (grade 1-2, 70% survival vs. grade 3-4, 54% survival) [1, 5, 6-10]. In a study of 315 patients Jalan emphasized how the immediate cause of death, for patients suffering from extremely serious hepatic damage, was in 35% of cases cerebral herniation secondary to intracranic hypertension. Untreatable, septic-shock-induced, secondary hypotension and multiple organ failure were the cause of death, or concurred to it, for a large part of the patients observed [7].

When encephalopathy, serious coagulopathy, acidosis and altered renal function dictate to contact and to transfer the patient to an approved specialised centre where it is possible to carry out an urgent liver transplant, there still are criteria arguing for the patient's admission to intensive care [1-12]. Hepatic encephalopathy rising from grade 2 to grade 3 is an assured criterium for intubation (airway protection when control is lost.) Haemodynamic instability, progressive and further worsening of haemostatic profile with possible thrombocytopenia (practically a DIC), acute respiratory insufficiency, acute renal insufficiency are also often but not always present and the scenario is that of MOF [1, 3-6, 10].

Prognostic criteria for paracetamol-induced and non-paracetamol-induced ALF are the same criteria currently adopted as urgent OLT indication (King's College Criteria; Table 4.4) [1, 4-8, 10, 18-22].

Today, prognostic criteria for paracetamol-induced ALF include, besides pH, coagulation profile, creatinine clearance and encephalopathy grade, also lactate clearance before or after volemic resuscitation (> 3,5-4 mEq/L). Lactate clearance as an indicator for prognosis and transplant timing remains however on the debating table [18-21]. An alternative to King's College criteria are the Clichy

Table 4.4 King's College criteria for urgent liver transplant indication [5]

Non paracetamol-induced ALF
INR >6.7
Or three of the following criteria:
Unfavourable aetiology (drugs, seronegativity)
Age <10 years or >40 years
Acute/sub-acute onset
Bilirubinemia above 18 mg/dL (300 mmol/L)
INR >3.5
Paracetamol-induced ALF
Arterial pH <7.3 post volemic resuscitation
Or concurrent reports of:
• Grade 3 or higher encephalopathy
• Creatinine clearance above 3.5 mg/dL (300 mmol)
• INR >6.5
• Lactate >3.5 mmol/L after 4 hours or >3 mmol/L after 12 hours

Criteria used in France to determine the indication for liver transplant and they are based on the degree of encephalopathy (grade 3 or 4) and on factor V level monitoring.

Factor V levels of < 20% for patients aged < 30 or < 30% for people aged > 30 [3-10, 22-25] represent the criteria for indicating that a liver transplant is urgent in the presence of ALF.

Intensive care management is optimal when linked to a Liver Transplant Centre and when it aims to support and to optimize vital functions [1, 4-7, 10] both in view of a liver transplant, if and when indicated, and with a view to combat or contain the onset of multiple organ failure (MOF) [1, 5, 6, 10]. In this context it is important to remember the role of N-acetyilcysteine (NAC) at high dose for the treatment of both paracetamol-induced ALF [1, 3-6, 10] and non-paracetamol-induced ALF [1, 26, 27]; early NAC treatment appears to be critical [1, 26, 27]. The scheme customarily used is a loading dose of 150 mg/kg for the first hour followed by 12,5 mg/kg for the next 4 hours and continuous IV infusion of 6.25 mg/kg for the remaining 67 hours (for a total of 72 hours of treatment) [26, 27]. The treatment, verified through a randomized trial, was associated with a higher no-transplant survival rate of the patients treated (40% vs. 27%; p = 0.043); the survival rate was in particular significantly higher in the subgroup with grade 1 and 2 encephalopathy (early stage) while it was equal for grade 3 and 4 encephalopathy. The authors came to the conclusion of adopting early NAC use in any case of ALF. NAC treatment does not appear to offer benefits for advanced stage coma that instead requires emergency OLT [1, 26, 27].

For the management of an ALF patient it is necessary to implement a comprehensive monitoring to target the multiple organ dysfunctions that normally follow [4-7, 10, 12]. Monitoring must therefore include checks on brain, heart, lungs and kidney function as well as on metabolic function (glycaemia and natraemia in particular), on coagulation profile and, if possible, on those coagulation factors which are included in the criteria that support the indication for urgent liver transplant. Currently, the Indocyanine Green test (PDR ICG clearance, LiMon Pulsion) [28-30] is also suggested particularly when monitoring liver function. History of ICG clearance testing is codified and documented in critical patients, in post-liver transplant stage and in hepatic resection (pre-surgery function evaluation; post-surgical function recovery) whereas in the ALF context this experience is limited. PDR ICG levels lower than 8-10% / minute are considered of pathological significance.

Extremely low levels do not necessarily invoke an inauspicious prognosis especially when associated to bilirubinemia levels > 6 mg/dL; bilirubin is in fact able to compete with the IGC carrier thus producing false positive results [31].

4.3   Central Nervous System Compromise: Monitoring and Treatment

It has been demonstrated that hepatic encephalopathy (see also Table 14.2) and cerebral oedema are linked to high levels of ammonia being generated in the hepatosplanchnic region and not being metabolized by the liver thus causing glutamine accumulation in brain astrocytes [7, 10, 32-37]. Ammoniaemia and glutamine concentration in the brain have been linked to intracranial pressure (ICP) level and to the onset of intracranial hypertension [33-37]. A raised ammonia level (> 124 mmol/L) has been linked to the onset of severe encephalopathy and to an unfavourable outcome and it is regarded as a specific and accurate parameter for prognosis [5, 6, 10, 34-37]. Hyponatraemia (< 125 mmol/L) and hyperglycaemia are two other metabolic factors that can affect the outcome [5, 6, 10]. EEG is used to monitor the CNS although it is not specific to this [32]. The progressive worsening of hepatic coma is characterised by a particular pattern of electrical brain activity showing a progressive slowdown and triphasic waves. (Fig. 4.2 and 4.3). EEG is indicated when there is a sudden encephalopathy alteration, when coma scale is 3-4 and when barbiturates are administered [4, 32].

Intracranic pressure (ICP) monitoring does not elicit unanimous consensus [5, 6, 10, 32, 87] nor can it improve outcome [87]. Less than 50% of the Transplant Centres have adopted this criterium. ICP level (to be maintained below 40 mmHg) allows targeted therapeutic intervention even though, as mentioned, it is not linked to a better outcome; increased morbidity (10-20%) and increased mortality (1-5%) are also reported. Prolonged periods of brain hypoperfusion with CPP < 50 mmHg or with ICP above 40 mmHg are linked to unfavourable outcome [4-7, 10, 32].

An indirect and less invasive way to monitor oxygen use and brain perfusion, but probably not as effective, is to measure jugular bulb oxygen saturation

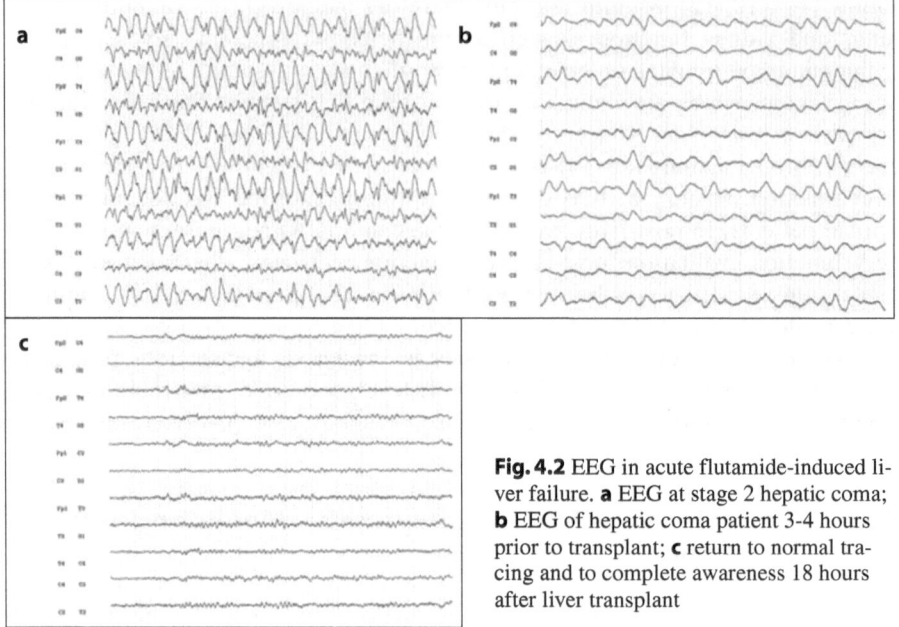

Fig. 4.2 EEG in acute flutamide-induced liver failure. **a** EEG at stage 2 hepatic coma; **b** EEG of hepatic coma patient 3-4 hours prior to transplant; **c** return to normal tracing and to complete awareness 18 hours after liver transplant

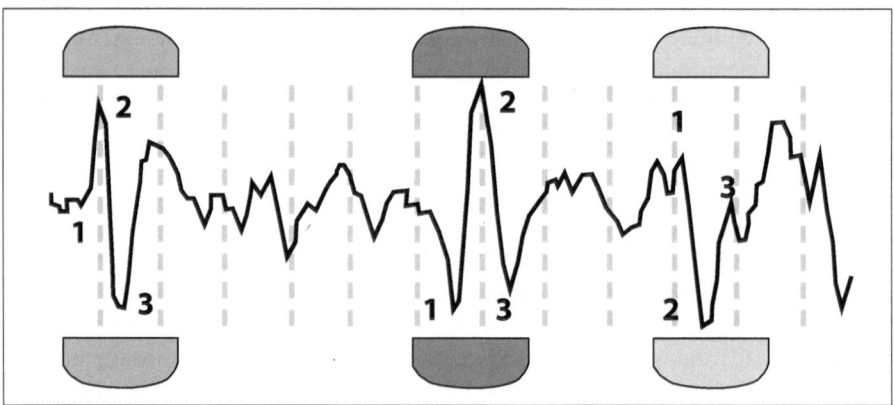

Fig. 4.3 EEG in flutamide-induced acute liver failure, triphasic waves (*magnification*)

(SjO$_2$) [5]. The use of transcranial Doppler [32] is extremely interesting; this type of imaging has reached an advanced phase of development. A few have recently proposed also optic nerve measurement by echography . Brain scans such as CAT, MRI and SPECT have, in this context, limited reliability; they present logistics difficulties and it is not always possible to carry out these procedures [5, 6].

In advanced-stage hepatic encephalopathy (3-4) it is important to minimize the risk of increased ICP; it is strongly recommended to raise the patient's head

(20°-30°), to intubate to protect the airway, to conduct controlled ventilation and to maintain adequate sedation levels (Propofol 3-5 mg/kg/hr) in order to reduce the state of agitation, concurrent metabolic surges, intracranial pressure and brain oxygen over-use [4-7, 10, 32]. Long-term maintenance includes also the administration of pentobarbital which a number of doctors use until a burst-suppression EEG is obtained [32].

Further measures are the maintenance of cardio-circulatory balance (to avoid hypotension), of normoxia and normocapnia (hyperventilation and hypocapnia do not appear to be necessary since they are only useful in treating unresponsive episodes of intracranic hypertension), mannitol administration to reduce brain oedema, normoglycaemia maintenance and frequent checks of sodium levels in order to avoid hyperosmolar syndrome [4-7, 10, 32].

Maintaining a state of low-moderate hypothermia (32-34° C) is of great relevance [4-7, 10, 32]. The most recent randomized trial on the benefits of hypothermia in the course of ALF, however, has not confirmed this as a necessity (Storze Larsen, unpublished data.) Despite observing that a temperature of < 33°C results in a greater reduction of ammonia production, the side effects of this level of hypothermia (modified coagulation, altered metabolism, greater susceptibility to infections) outweigh potential advantages; a temperature range of 34-36°C is therefore recommended [1, 6].

Maintenance of brain perfusion pressure must be evaluated also in relation to systemic hypotension. Noradrenaline is the vasopressor usually administered in view of the haemodynamics profile (*vide infra*) [5, 6, 10, 32]. Terlipressin has been proposed in some cases but its use may result in increased intracranial pressure due to increased cerebral blood flow. Recent experience [4-7, 38] however contradicts what has been so far indicated thus removing the contraindication to terlipressin during the course of ALF. Eefesen [38] has in fact observed increased cerebral blood flow but no modification of intracranic pressure and also signs of restoration of blood flow autoregulation and absence of cerebral cell toxicity (evaluated through cerebral microdialysis for lactate and lactate/pyruvate ratio.)

4.4   Cardiovascular Compromise: Monitoring and Treatment

The cardiocirculatory profile of a patient with acute liver failure is defined by hyperkinetic syndrome, elevated cardiac index (often over 5 L/min/m^2), low mean arterial pressure, low systemic and pulmonary vascular resistance (under 600-800 dynes/s/cm^{-5}) and medium-low cardiac filling pressure. Increased cardiac output is sustained both by increased systolic output and by increased heart rate [4-7, 10] although the latter is not always present.

Vasodilation in the initial stages of ALF, as seen in kidneys and muscles, is linked to increased release and failed clearance of cytokines by the liver, reflecting a SIRS event [5]. There is a significant neuroendocrine response that in the later stages leads to a reduction of regional blood flow mediated by vasoconstriction [7] (Table 4.5). In the later stages the relevant mediators appear to be NO and cGMP; the origin of massive initial dilation is instead not yet completely understood [7].

The heart pumping function is almost always maintained and signs of heart failure are only evident in the final stages when they are likely linked to prolonged hypotension. Heart rhythm changes (bradyarrhythmia, AV block of various degree, ectopic beats and supraventricular tachyarrhythmia) or ST tract alterations appear to be linked to hypossia, hypovolemia or cerebral oedema and not to inherent cardiac disease or to liver failure per se. A massive systemic vasodilation frequently causes relative hypovolemia and it is the most frequent cause of hypotension observed in the course of ALF. Maintaining a balanced circulation requires the administration of fluids and, subsequently, of amines [4-7, 10]. Volemic replacement is accomplished via crystalloids and colloids and is mandated by filling pressure values (PVC) and eventually by ScvO$_2$ or, better, by methods that monitor cardiac output and SvO$_2$.

continuously as well by means of a modified Swan Ganz catheter or by volume assessment methods (PiCCO Pulsion, EV 1000 Edwards) that allow monitoring of intrathoracic blood volume (ITBVi) and extravascular lung water (EVLWi). ALF guidelines share the common target of maintaining a mean arterial pressure (MAP) of between 55 and 65 mmHg in order to both achieve adequate brain perfusion and to avoid hyper-afflux risk [4-7, 10].

Volumetric preload parameters have long shown to be more reliable than the classical pressure parameters, despite the latter being commonly suggested and used for the purpose of optimizing pressure, with due consideration to the complexity of ALF hypotension.

Fluid challenge and dynamic parameters of fluid responsiveness such as stroke volume variation (SVV) and pulse pressure variation (PPV) during controlled ventilation are certainly the preferred choice [4-7, 10, 39]. Interesting predictors of hypovolemia could be passive leg raising and correlated haemodynamic alterations even in non-ventilated patients. Echography could confirm inferior vena cava diameter. Vasoconstrictors administration (noradrenaline 0,1-0,7 g/kg/min or terlipressin if no response to noradrenaline) is suggested after having

Table 4.5 Cardiovascular profile in ALF and in chronic liver disease

	Acute liver failure	Advanced cirrhosis
Systemic Vascular Resistance	⇩⇩⇩	⇩⇩
Cardiac Output	⇧⇧⇧	⇧⇧
Mean Arterial Pressure	⇩⇩⇩	⇩/⇩⇩
Muscle blood flow	⇩⇧	⇩
Renal blood flow	⇩⇧	⇩
Splanchnic blood flow	⇧	⇧⇧
Critical hypotension and vascular collapse	++	*/-

Source: Jalan [7]; modified

optimized circulatory volume while performing at least simplified haemodynamic monitoring, i.e. invasive arterial blood pressure, central venous pressure and
ScvO2, (eventually also vaCO2) measurements which are today mandatory. Cardiac
output monitoring, mandatory in the presence of hypotension of difficult interpretation, invokes a methodology for the determination of cardiac output by
transpulmonary thermodilution (PiCCO Pulsion, EV 1000 Edwards) by means of
calibrated devices (LiDCOPlus) or Swan Ganz catheter [4, 5, 6, 39]. Cardiac output assessment through minimally invasive techniques (arterial pressure wave-
form analysis: Vigileo FlowTrack, LiDCOrapid, PRAM as self-calibrated methods) has not yet been validated for hyperkinetic syndrome with elevated cardiac
output despite the most recent data arguing in favour of the latest version Vigileo
Flow Track's reliability [89, 90]. Transthoracic echocardiogram is a useful tool to
evaluate heart's contractility, even if only by sight, and pericardial effusion.
Ventricular chamber filling (by sight), IVC diameter and its changes in patients
under controlled ventilation are further data to be examined in order to reach a
diagnosis of volemic state and to optimize such state [39]. Despite its current
infrequent use, echocardiography could be useful considering that in ALF there
is also a not yet fully understood increase of troponin I levels [40]. Recent data
argue in favour of latent adrenal insufficiency that responds to steroid treatment
(but some hold the opinion that adrenal insufficiency must be confirmed by short
sinachten test). A dosage of 200-300 mg OD of hydrocortisone for 5-7 days
allowed for noradrenaline dose reduction during ALF (Identical effect to that
observed during severe sepsis/septic shock.) It is in any case suggested by some
that hydrocortisone be administered to those patients with hypotension that is
resistant to fluids and to noradrenaline [4-7, 10, 41].

4.5 Respiratory Compromise: Monitoring and Treatment

Invasive haemodynamic monitoring facilitates also the evaluation of acute
hypoxemic respiratory failure which often (40%) accompanies ALF and frequently includes interstitial pulmonary oedema (Fig. 4.4) [4-7, 10, 42, 81].
Monitoring includes, in this case, besides EVLWi after PiCCO or EV 1000 positioning, also haemogas analysis and radiological imaging (X-ray and/or CAT
and /or thoracic echography.)
    Thoracic ultrasound is an interesting application in this context. Ventilation
must be conducted with regard to recent procedures of protective ventilation
considering nonetheless the need to avoid hypercapnia. In practice the procedure
would require: TV 6-8 mL/kg; plateau pressure 30 cmH2O; PEEP 8-10 cmH2O
(which is optimized after alveolar recruitment manoeuvre by appropriate methods) and adequate respiratory frequency to maintain normocapnia, as previously observed on the subject of brain perfusion [4-7, 10, 32, 42-45, 81]. Invasive
diagnostic and therapeutic procedures such as bronchoscopy – for evaluating
bronchial obstruction or to carry out a BAL – and non-invasive procedures such
as thoracic echography [46] – for evaluating interstitial oedema through B lines,

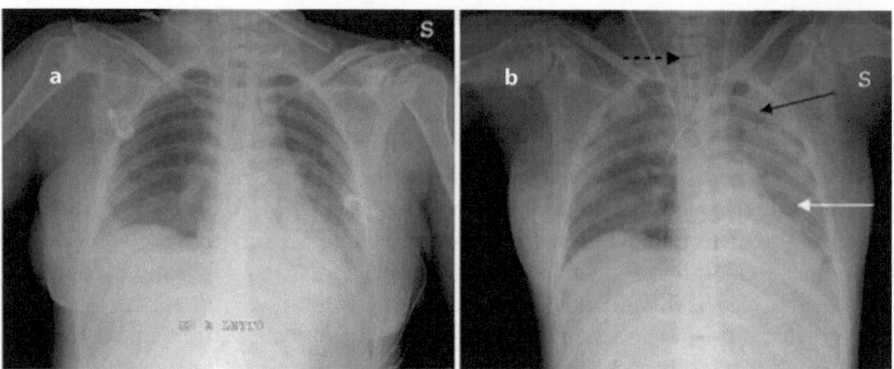

Fig. 4.4 a Rapid evolution interstitial oedema in a patient with viral hepatitis B -induced FHF (fulminant hepatic failure). **b** Continuous haemofiltration (*black arrow*), Swan Ganz catheter (*white arrow*) and endotracheal tube (*dotted arrow*)

pleural effusion, atelectasis or dysventilation areas with subsequent fibrobron-choscopy – are today important tools for a comprehensive diagnosis of respira-tory insufficiency. The possible role of increased intra-abdominal pressure in relation to thoracic symptoms must finally be considered. It is therefore suggest-ed to monitor abdominal pressure [4-7, 10, 47].

4.6   Renal Compromise: Monitoring and Treatment

Renal insufficiency is present in 40-70% of cases: incidence variability often depends on the ambiguous definition [4-7, 10, 48, 81]. The causes are multiple and the physiopathology is complex. According to O'Grady there is a combina-tion of a functional condition similar to hepatorenal syndrome and of acute tubu-lar necrosis [12]. Absolute or, more frequently, relative hypovolemia [1, 4-7, 10, 12, 48, 81] is often concurrent to renal hypoperfusion secondary to systemic vasodilation and to selective renal vasoconstriction (Table 4.3). The monitoring process includes hourly diuresis and urine electrolytes (chloriduria is interest-ing, as reported in [92]; it also relies on haemodynamic profile interpretation (as revealed by both minimally invasive monitoring devices and others such as SG, PiCCO or EV 100), on static or dynamic devices to optimize volemia and on an indirect evaluation of renal perfusion pressure (see above). The measurement of renal perfusion pressure must take into consideration inferior vena cava and intra-abdominal pressure – subtracted from mean arterial pressure; this step allows clinicians to gather information on abdominal hypertension (present at > 16 mmHg), a condition that may cause significant modifications to renal perfu-sion pressure [47]. Ascites, abdominal wall or intestinal oedema are contribut-ing conditions to an abdominal compartment syndrome; haemoperitoneum may be present in some rare cases [4-7, 10, 47].

Treatment consists first of all in optimizing volemia (see above), then in sensible administration of diuretics (furosemide, ethacrynic acid, mannitol) and vasopressors (usually noradrenaline to increase glomerular perfusion pressure) [4-7, 10, 32]. Although terlipressin is justified in the presence of hepatorenal syndrome associated to chronic liver insufficiency [49-51], its use lacks sufficient corroboration in the ALF context [5] despite the fact that recent information, previously and already reviewed, modifies these statements [6, 38]. The renal effect of terlipressin is mediated by V_1 receptors at splanchnic level enabling selective vasoconstriction of the efferent renal arteriole and increased glomerular filtration pressure. The cerebral effect is instead mediated by V_2 receptors resulting in vasodilation with increased cerebral blood flow and intracranial pressure and therefore also increased risk of cerebral oedema [5, 49-51]. Continuous renal replacement therapy (CRRT) is preferred to intermittent therapy due to its better cardiocirculatory tolerance and its constant and continuous effect. It must be initiated early and it is an integral part of the treatment aimed at reducing cerebral oedema [4-7, 10]; there are no full-standard criteria and recently there has been some perplexity on the subject. The current reinfusion parameters are approximately 30-35 mL/kg/hr [52, 53]. Bicarbonate-based solutions are the preferred choice for reinfusion [5, 6, 10] given the inability of a failing liver to metabolize lactate and the consequent difficulty in evaluating its levels. When thrombocytopenia and serious coagulation deficit are present, the use of prostacyclin as anticoagulant is interesting (Epoprostenol Sodium, 2-6 ng/kg/min) [4-7, 10, 54]. The recent experience of high volume exchange techniques (HVE, 90 mL/kg/hr) appears to be promising but such techniques are very demanding at clinical and nursing level and are still at experimental stage [6]. No evidence supports the use of either dopamine (even if it has been re-proposed recently) or fenoldopam.

4.7   Infections: Monitoring and Treatment

The patient with acute liver failure is particularly susceptible to infection, especially bacterial infections (> 70% Gram-positive cocci, Gram-negative bacilli) and mycotic infections (> 30% and increased incidence of Aspergillus spp-induced infections) [4-7, 10, 55-59]. There is in fact a reduction in both opsonization capability (reduced complement levels) and macrophage phagocytic function (paralysis of histiocytic reticular system of which the liver has a high content) [58]. Central catheter-related infections of the respiratory and urinary tract and bacterial infections are reported most frequently. Survival decreases when SIRS and/or proven infections are present [4-7, 55-59]. It is therefore important to have infectiology monitoring protocol guidelines for optimal use of antibiotics and antifungal drugs (Candida colonization index, or Candida score that identifies colonizations at risk of becoming invasive infections is very interesting in this respect) [60]. Systemic treatment with antibiotics (third-generation cephalosporins) possibly combined with selective gastroenteric decontamination has shown to be effective in lowering the incidence of sepsis and improving hepatic encephalopathy grade but there has been no clear sign of any effect on the outcome [59]. Chlorexidine for oral hygiene is another possible way to reduce oral cavity colonization and VAP [61, 62].

Prophylactic antibiotic treatment is not recommended. New American guidelines [10] and the most recent review of this problem instead suggest empirical antibacterial and antifungal treatment when the situation is such that urgent liver transplant is considered or if sepsis risk is high; such risk manifests itself with the onset of SIRS, the identification of micro-organisms in monitoring cultures, the progression towards 3-4 encephalopathy and the onset of refractory hypotension. To date no recommendation based on adequate evidence is available with regard to the choice of antibiotics or antifungal drugs. It is however imperative to take into consideration monitoring cultures, department and hospital ecology and patients' risk factors [5, 6, 10]. Pharmacokinetics and pharmacodynamics criteria as well as the above-mentioned microbiological criteria must in any case be considered today as the priority that dictates the choice of anti-infective drugs in this context [63, 64].

4.8   Haemostatic Profile Alterations: Monitoring and Treatment

ALF includes severe coagulopathy (PT-INR > 1.5 although > 5 is not infrequent) while the presence of thrombocytopenia or thrombocytopathy [10, 65-67] is variable. Coagulation factors (except for VIII) and natural anticoagulant factors are synthesized in the liver so there is an unbalance of various degree between procoagulant and anticoagulant factors. The gravity of coagulatory alterations is associated to the aetiology of ALF, in the presence of prolonged INR for instance when the symptoms reflect hepatitis B-induced fulminant liver failure [65]. Reduced synthesis of coagulation factors (in particular of Vitamin K-dependent types II, VII, IX, X and V), their increased use by the body, a reduced clearance of activated coagulation factors and their inhibitors (a condition associated to reticuloendothelial system dysfunction) all contribute to define an altered haemostasis. The short half-life of factors V and VII causes the rapid changes in coagulation tests and also confirms their importance in ALF syndrome [23-25].

Some clinicians maintain that a reduced degradation of natural anticoagulants is also present [65, 66]. The clinical signs can in this case be likened to those of a DIC of thrombotic nature at first but becoming haemorrhagic later. Differential diagnosis between DIC and hyperfibrinolysis can be very difficult. The presence of microthrombi at organ level (e.g. kidneys) is usually associated with DIC while normal AT and Factor VIII levels and absence of microthrombi suggest fibrinolysis [63]. The presence of fibrinolysis in ALF is in fact controversial because a significant increase in tissue plasminogen activator (tPA), associated to a state of hyperfibrinolysis, is sometimes concurrent with an even

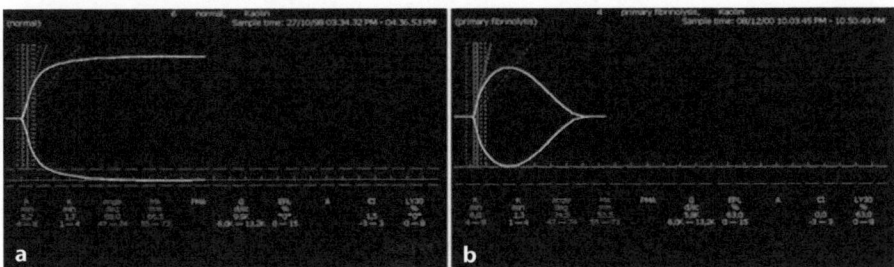

Fig. 4.5 Thromboelastography trace (TEG). **a** Normal tracing, **b** hyperfibrinolysis tracing

greater increase of plasminogen activator inhibitor 1 (PAI-1) which can in turn lead to hypofibrinolysis [65]. Hyperfibrinolysis (confirmed by the presence of D-dimer and other fibrin degradation products or by thromboelastography findings) causes procoagulant factors inhibition and tendency to bleeding (Fig. 4.5).

Fibrin degradation products binding with platelet fibronogen receptors (integrin IIb-3) may itself be the cause of platelet aggregation inhibition and of bleeding [65].

Optimal management of ALF-related coagulopathy identifies some established standpoints while others are still under discussion and therefore in need of proof by evidence. At the forefront there is the necessity, not yet proven, to supplement antithrombin [4-7, 10, 65, 67]. Spontaneous bleeding is not frequent and yet it is possible to gather records of an approximate 30% incidence of major haemorrhaging [65]. The most recent guidelines [4-7, 10, 65-66] discourage prophylactic use of replacement therapy with fresh-frozen plasma (FFP), platelets and cryoprecipitates. Recent experience shows evidence, however, of a general tendency to administer FFP and platelets, a treatment that produces short-term haemostasis, a risk of volume overload, transfusion related acute lung injury (TRALI) and increased cerebral oedema [65-66]. It is instead recommended to administer FFP (15-20 mL/kg), platelets (one platelet concentrate per 10 kg body weight) and cryoprecipitates when fibrinogen level < 100 mg/dL in case of significant bleeding taking place or for patients undergoing invasive procedures [10, 60-65, 81]. A possible alternative is the use of prothrombin complex concentrate despite its administration giving rise to uncertainty due to its role in potentially activating coagulation. Diagnostics should dictate administration which should be based both on static tests (PT/INR, aPTT, fibrinogenemia, platelet count, D-dimer) and dynamic investigations such as thromboelastography. FFP, platelets and cryoprecipitates may in this context be administered according to parameters that can pinpoint each single need [68].

Plasmapheresis has always been given consideration but its usefulness has never been proven and its use to treat coagulopathy is currently uncommon. Recorded experience on this subject is anecdotal; it is related to paediatrics and based on work by Asian teams [65, 69]. The use of antifibrinolytic agents is proposed by some but there is a lack of substantial logic to such use despite their administration having shown, in some cases, a reduction of or an end to bleeding [65, 66]. The role of recombinant activated agent VII (Novoseven, Novo) is also reported as promising especially prior to risky invasive procedures or prior to transplant surgery [65, 66, 70]. Dosage and administration method have yet to be established; in particular it is still under discussion whether PFC or platelet administration must be undertaken before administering agent VII [70]. Prophylactic administration has not produced any results [65, 66]. Vitamin K parenteral administration, in the course of ALF, excludes its deficiency as the basic cause of a coagulation pathology [66].

4.9   Artificial Hepatic Support

As it has been so far pointed out, ALF produces a very serious alteration of all hepatic functions: protein synthesis, excretion, depuration and metabolic functions. Glycogenolysis and gluconeogenesis suffer alterations and the synthesis of coagulation factors, of physiological anticoagulants and of proteins including albumin is reduced [1-12].

Bilirubin, aromatic amino acids, bile salts, endogenous benzodiazepines, prostacyclin, tryptophan, nitric oxide are some of the many substances previously mentioned that are bound to and/or carried by albumin. It is deemed that all these substances, since there is an increase in their free level and a reduced excretion, are the concurrent cause of multiple organ failure in the course of ALF. While conventional dialysis methods are acceptable for the removal of hydrophilic substances, the substances bound to albumin require a special adsorber or acceptor [1, 6, 10, 71-75]. Intensive care of an ALF patient can today rely on artificial support, that is still being developed, and that may be used, in the interim, both as a bridge to transplant and as a support to spontaneous liver regeneration [71-82]. It is however important to clarify [1, 74] right at this point that extracorporeal treatment alone currently holds insufficient evidence to be considered as an alternative to transplant.

There are two types of support: artificial and bioartificial support [75]. Artificial (acellular) support originates from haemodialysis, a procedure used since the very beginning that has however only achieved a modest ammonia reduction thus confirming insignificant results. There has been no change of outcome even when using haemoperfusion with adsorbent substances (carbon, resins) despite some positive results in animal experimentation; in fact neither ammonia nor albumin-bound toxins were adequately removed and there were also problems with platelet aggregation and release of vasoactive substances [71, 72, 75]. Plasmapheresis has not produced univocal results despite being successful in a few, especially paediatric, cases [69].

A system, unfolding through several phases, is the combination of haemodiafiltration, haemoperfusion with carbon and the use of cation-exchange resins. Such system has shown to remove toxins up to 5000 D and also some albumin-bound toxins. Even this method however, despite the most recent innovations, has not produced any significant results on the outcome. Some studies have reported a neurological improvement [72]. The most recent, and currently most used, methods require the use of albumin as scavenger molecule as it can bind (acceptor or adsorber) toxic molecules which are often hydrosoluble but are most frequently bound to albumin and therefore non hydrosoluble, as previously mentioned [71, 75]. Albumin dialysis is a high-flux detoxifying treatment where albumin is used as dialysis solution along with high permeability membranes. Blood toxins are eliminated by diffusion and bound to dialysate albumin. Devices currently on the market are: MARS (Molecular Adsorbent Recirculating System, Teraklin Gambro) [75, 78], SPAD (Single Pass Albumin Dialysis) [78] and Prometheus (Fresenius) [79].

The MARS device, object of most of the studies and the oldest on the market, consists of a blood circuit, an albumin circuit and a "kidney" circuit [73, 75-77]. The patient's blood is circulated in a hollow-fiber polysulfone membrane haemodialyzer. The membrane is albumin-coated with < 50-60 kDa cut off in order to avoid loss of endogenous albumin, hormones, growth factors and carrier proteins. Dialysate consists of a continous flow of 20% albumin circulating in the extracapillary compartment. Its use as dialysis agent is dictated by its ability to bind molecules normally carried by albumin. The membrane acts as adsorber for albumin-bound toxins and the same toxins are subsequently picked up by dialysate albumin which then passes through haemodialysis or haemofiltration. Hydrosoluble molecules and protein-bound toxins are removed immediately, as soon as they bind to albumin on one side of the filtering membrane and subsequently when they bind to countercurrent albumin on the opposite side of the filtering membrane. Albumin is then passed through a carbon filter for regeneration and finally through a dialyser to remove urea and creatinine.

Despite the very optimistic initial reports on MARS potentiality in modifying ALF-related multiple organ failure syndrome (haemodynamics profile and neurological state improvement, in some cases also improvement of coagulation as well as ammonia, bilirubin and lactate reduction) there is to date no evidence that MARS alters mortality rates when used for treating ALF especially if short-term urgent liver transplant is not possible [73, 74, 75]. The experience is limited to small groups. In a study of randomized patients undergoing MARS or standard treatment, there were no significant changes of outcome despite the presence of significant alterations in the haemodynamic profile. Reported cases of identical experiences confirm modifications of metabolism and circulation but no effect on the outcome [74, 75].

SPAD is instead a simpler technique using conventional machines for CRRT in CVVHD and a hollow-fiber high-flux dialysis module without the added system of pumps and recycling modules [78]. The albumin solution (1000 mL albumin 20% in 3500 mL of dialysate) is circulated in countercurrent flow. Protein-bound and hydrosoluble substances pass through the albumin-rich membrane and are eliminated by diffusion. The albumin solution is in turn eliminated after passing through the filter. A recent in-vitro comparison study of MARS and SPAD has confirmed SPAD's identical detoxifying capability which has proved to be effective and probably cost-effective as well [78].

Prometheus System (Fresenius Medical Care AG) [79, 80] is another system based on a variation of albumin dialysis, plasma separation and adsorbtion via high-flux dialysis. A very recent review on the subject has in fact considered this system, when properly indicated, as a most interesting option able to increase survival possibility for ALF patients awaiting transplant [75, 80].

Even the most recent reviews on the subject of artificial support in the course of ALF cannot confirm a change of outcome [74, 7].

Bioartificial or hybrid support requires the use of freshly-harvested or cryop-reserved human or porcine liver cells [75, 80].

Bioartificial systems (BAL, ELAD) consist of a bioreactor with a hollow fiber capillaries chamber; hollow fibers are loaded with human or porcine hepa-tocytes of varied matrix; the patient's plasma is passed through the fibers after having been separated, oxygenated and warmed. Molecule exchange happens through a semipermeable membrane of sufficient porosity and size to allow the passage of toxins and protein carriers (albumin, 66kD) involved in the onset of ALF but not that of immunoglobulins (100-900 kD), complement (200 kD), virus or cells (a source of great difficulty). Hepatocytes, deemed to be effective in a range between 6 and $36 \cdot 10^9$, extract oxygen and nutrients and remove tox-ins from plasma. Cell metabolites are returned to plasma.

The most advanced systems include carbon columns placed in front of the bioreactor in order to remove toxins that could damage porcine liver cells or else a detoxification module which would allow albumin dialysis and haemodiafiltra-tion (MELS, using human hepatocytes from livers obtained from cadaver donors and deemed unsuitable for transplant).

Problems linked to the type of cells used are zoonosis in case of porcine cells (but to date there is no evidence of this occurrence and the method is therefore to be considered extremely safe) and cancer cell seeding of prototypes as prac-ticed in the late 90s using hepatoblastoma cells [75, 80].

Data gathered through randomized studies taking place up until now are pos-itive when considered individually or within a case report (neurological profile improvement, intracranial pressure reduction) but fail to prove a significant reduction in mortality through the use of artificial support [75, 81]. The most comprehensive study published on the use of BAL (HepatAssist Arbios, USA) in ALF patients with fulminant or sub-fulminant hepatitis on a liver transplant list and patients with post-transplant primary non-function randomized to receive both standard treatment and BAL has confirmed the same survival rate in the group that was treated (73%) and in the control group (73 vs 62%, ns). Treated patient showed a greater tendency to survival. In a post-hoc analysis the study highlighted a significantly higher survival rate (44%, $p < 0,048$) of patients with fulminant or sub-fulminant liver failure of known aetiology treated with artificial support versus the patients suffering from unknown cause ALF [81, 91]. A study is taking place with a boosted version of HepatAssist (20 billion porcine cells compared to 7,5 billion in the original version) [91].

The most recent Cochrane review on ALF treatment by means of artificial or bioartificial extracorporeal support versus standard treatment does not highlight any advantage in relation to mortality (RR 0.86; 95% CI 0.65 - 1.12) or in the bridge to urgent liver transplant (RR 0.87; 95% CI 0.73 - 1.05) while an improvement of hepatic encephalopathy (RR 0.67; 95% CI 0.52 - 0.86) is noted. A positive effect is reported on mortality in cases of MARS-treated acute-on-chronic liver failure (RR 0.67; 95% CI 0.51 - 0.90) [74].

4.10   Liver Transplant

Emergency liver transplant is today a routine procedure in many European countries and in North America. Liver transplant has changed fulminant hepatitis prognosis [1, 9, 91]. Despite the survival rate being higher for elective transplant than for emergency transplant due to multiple organ failure complications in the latter, the rate for patients who had an emergency transplant is today close to 80%. The factors that determine the outcome are indication accuracy and timing and possible presence of associated pathologies that could compromise the results of a surgical technique that is today quite sophisticated (85% one-year survival in Italy, Centro Nazionale Trapianti February 2011). An accurate and early indication is certainly one of the most crucial factors. As previously stated, transplant indication criteria include some of the factors which have proved to be significant in affecting ALF mortality in absence of transplant: encephalopathy grade, age, liver compromise severity (bilirubin level) and degree of coagulation changes. King's College criteria, certainly the most referred to for emergency transplant indication, include also ALF's cause and symptom manifestations while Clichy criteria take into account besides encephalopathy grade also factor V level and age [1]. These criteria are sufficiently specific; in fact, the survival rate for non-transplanted patient who meet such criteria requirements is <15%. Sensitivity however may not be satisfactory; such criteria are unable to identify certain patients who would die if they did not undergo emergency transplant. For the purpose of increasing sensitivity it has been suggested that some variables be introduced (MELD, lactate, phosphate levels, alpha-Fetoprotein). They have however failed to significantly increase performance. A revision of the criteria is very likely in the near future [1]. It would be useful for scores and point scales to have high predicting power with regard to survival without transplant (positive outcome further to standard treatment alone) and not just with regard to mortality without transplant. Present criteria forecast mortality but not survival [84]. The most recent and undoubtedly interesting proposal is to also use MELD and replace bilirubin value with cell death marker CK18/M65, one of the cytoskeleton protein family intermediate filaments.

Early experience shows M65 value to be linked to the absence of cell vitality spontaneous recovery. This marker seems therefore able to predict cell death and absence of spontaneous functional recovery [85].

It is in any case a certainty that emergency transplant outcome is greatly influenced by several factors: the recipient's age (recipient mortality doubles when age > 50), the seriousness of a patient's pre-transplant condition and the graft quality. Despite lack of confirmation for every single case, steatosis > 40-50% is associated with failed or very poor functional recovery [1]. A considerable problem is whether to accept a sub-optimal or "marginal" graft (known today as extended criteria donor graft) which statistically is likely to produce a worse outcome but that is readily available or wait for a better quality liver that may however arrive too late [1]. Asian practice, given the nearly total lack of cadaver donors, allows also emergency liver transplant from living donor. In this case, the ethical problem stems from a conflict between evaluating suitability and performing a right hepatectomy on a healthy donor who does not need any intervention and least of all with any urgency. This procedure is reported as having a donor mortality rate between 0.3 and 0.5% and a morbidity rate of 15 to 50%. The most recent data show a recipient survival rate close to 80% (from cadaver donor survival varies between 50 and 75%) [91]. The hypothesis of extracorporeal artificial or bioartificial replacement, as previously mentioned, cannot thus be considered the sole possibility for support. The same consideration is valid for hepatocyte transplant despite the report of interesting case results and of related anecdotal literature [1].

4.11 Conclusions

ALF, a syndrome presenting acute hepatic encephalopathy and seriously altered coagulation, despite significant improvements in the treatment, still carries a high mortality rate, it requires early diagnosis, a complex multi-disciplinary treatment and recognizes liver transplant as the only therapeutic option able to modify its outcome. All the adopted measures (top intensive care, use of artificial or bioartificial methods) must be aimed at facilitating liver function spontaneous recovery, when possible, or at allowing a bridge to transplant. There are coded criteria that indicate urgent liver transplant in the presence of ALF. Cerebral function deterioration (coma progression from grade 2 to 3) suggests an indication for observation and top intensive care along with contact with a Transplant Centre for a possible protected transferral of the patient. Coma progression to grade 3 mandates protective intubation. Early and constant contact with Intensive Care doctors, surgeons and Transplant Centres' hepatologists allows for diagnostic and therapeutic measures to be put in place and to be directed towards containing multi organ failure and establishing a prompt indication for liver transplant [86, 92]. Artificial or bioartificial replacement methods, although promising in the ALF context, represent to date measures for support until emergency transplant is achieved. Further improvement in the outcome of this rare but extremely serious pathology is undoubtedly dependent on identifying ALF at an increasingly earlier stage and on establishing a targeted treatment. Improving indication criteria could also further increase survival [1, 86].

Bibliografia

1. Bernal W, Auzinger G, Dhawan A , Wendon J (2010) Acute liver failure. Lancet 376:190-201
2. Grady JC, Schalm SW, Williams R (1993) Acute liver failure: redifining the syndrome. Lancet 342: 273-275
3. Lee WM (2003) Acute liver failure in USA. Sem Liver Dis 23: 217-226
4. Trotter JF (2009) Practical management of acute liver failure in the intensive care unit. Curr Op Crit Care15:163-167
5. Stravitz RT (2008) Critical management decisions in patirnts with acute liver failure. Chest 134;1092-1102
6. Auzinger G, Wedon J (2008) Intensive care management of acute hepatic failure. Curr Op Crit Care 14:179-188
7. Jalan R (2005) Acute liver failure: current management and future perspects. J Hepatol 42: S115-S123
8. Ichai P, Samuel D (2008) Etiology and prognosis of fulminant hepatitis in adults. Liver Transplantation 14:S67-S79
9. Bernal W, Wendon J (2004) Liver transplantation in adults with acute liver failure. J Hepatol 40: 192-197
10. Stravitz RT, Kramer AH, Davern T et al (2007) Intensive care of patients with acute liver failure: recommendations of the US Acute Liver Failure Study Group. Crit Care Med 35:2498-2508
11. Ostapowicz G, Fontana RJ, Schiødt FV et al (2002) Results of a prospective study of acute liver failure at 17 tertiary care centers in the United States. Ann Intern Med 137:947-954
12. O'Grady JG (2005) Acute liver failure. Postgrad Med J 81:148-154
13. Khashab M , Tector J, Kwo PJ (2007) Epidemiology of acute liver failure. Current Gastroenterology Reports 9:66-73
14. De Carlis L, De Gasperi A et al (2001) Liver transplantation for ecstasy induced fulminant hepatic failure. Transpl Proc 33:2743-2744
15. Munoz SJ, Reddy RK, Lee W (2008) The coagulopathy of acute liver failure and implications for intracranial pressure monitoring. Neurocrit Care 9:103-107
16. Lisman T, Leebeek F (2007) Hemostatic alterations in liver disease: a review on pathophysiology, clinical consequences, and treatment. Dig Surg 24:250-258
17. De Gasperi A, Corti A, Mazza E et al (2009) Acute liver failure: managing coagulopathy and the bleeding diathesis. Transpl Proc 41:1256-1259
18. O'Grady JC, Alexander GJ, Hayllar KM, Williams R (1989) Early predictors of prognosis in fulminant hepartic failure. Gastroenterology 97:439-445
19. Bernal W, Donaldson N, Wyncoll D, Wendon J (2002) Blood lactate as an early predictor of outcome in paracetamol-induced acute liver failure: a cohort study. Lancet 358:558-563
20. Riordan SM, William R (2003) Mechanisms of hepatic injury, multiorgan failure and prognostic criteria in ALF. Sem Liver Dis 23:204-215
21. Schmidt LE, Larsen FS (2006) Prognostic implications of hyperlactatemia, multiple organ failure and systemic inflammatory response syndrome in patients with acetaminophen-induced acute liver failure. Crit Care Med 34:337-343
22. Devlin J, O'Grady J (1999) Indications for referral and assessment in adult liver transplantation: a clinical guideline. Gut 45(Suppl VI):1-22
23. Elinav E, Ben-Dov I, Hai-Am E et al (2005) The predictive value of admission and follow-up factor V and VII levels in patients with acute hepatitis and coagulopathy. J Hepatol 42: 82-86
24. Bernuau J, Goudeau A, Poynard T et al (1986) Multivariate analysis of prognostic factors in fulminant hepatitis B. Hepatology 6:648-651
25. Bernuau J, Samuel D, Durand F et al (1991) Criteria for emergency liver transplantation in patients with acute viral hepatitis and factor V below 50% of normal: A prospective study. Abstr Hepatology 14:49A

26. Lee WM et al (2009) Intravenous n-acetylcysteine improves transplant-free survival in early stage non-acetaminophen acute liver failure. Gastroenterology 137:856-864
27. Riordan SM, Williams R (2010) Management of non-acetaminophen-induced ALF. Nat Rev Gastroenterol Hepatol 7: 75-77
28. Jalan R, Plevris JN, Jalan QR et al (1994) A pilot study of indocyanine green as an early predictor of graft function. Transplantation58:196-200
29. Hetz H, Ploechl W, Berlakovich GA et al (2001) Intraoperative indocyanine green kinetics predict postoperative graft function after OLT for chronic hepatic failure. Am J Transplantation 1(Suppl 1):313
30. Hetz H, Faibyk P, Baker A et al (2002) Non invasive detection of ICG kinetics in OLT. Intensive Care Med 28:S1
31. Mazza E, Prosperi M, De Gasperi A et al (2008) PDR ICG after liver transplantation: always a reliable tool to predict graft function and outcome? Liver Transplantation 14:476
32. Frontera JA, Kalb T (2010) Neurological management of fulminant hepatic failure. Neurocrit Care. doi: 10.1007/s12028-010-9470-y
33. Vaquero J, Chung C, Cahill ME, Blei AT (2003) Pathogenesis of hepatic encephalopathy in acute liver failure. Sem Liver Dis 23: 259-269
34. Tofteng F, Hauerberg J, Hansen BA et al (2006) Persistent arterial hyperammonemia increases the concentration of glutamine and alanine in the brain and correlates with intracranial pressure in patients with fulminant hepatic failure. J Cereb Blood Flow Metab 26:21-27
35. Bhatia V, Singh R, Acharya SK (2006) Predictive value of arterial ammonia for complications and outcome in acute liver failure. Gut 55:98-104
36. Bernal W, Hall C, Karvellas CJ et al (2007) Arterial ammonia and clinical risk factors for encephalopathy and intracranial hypertension in acute liver failure. Hepatology 46:1844-1852
37. Jalan R (2003) Intracranial hypertension in ALF: pathophysiological basis of rational management. Sem Liver Dis 23: 271-282
38. Eefsen M, Dethloff T, Frederiksen HJ (2007) Comparison of terlipressin and noradrenalin on cerebral perfusion, intracranial pressure and extracellular concentrations of lactate and pyruvate in patients with acute liver failure in need of inotropic support. J Hepatol 47:381-386
39. Pinsky MR, Payen D (2005) Functional hemodynamic monitoring. Crit Care 9: 566-572
40. Parekh NK, Hynan LS, De Lemos J et al (2007) Elevated troponin I levels in acute liver failure: is myocardial injury an integral part of acute liver failure? Hepatology 45:1489-1495
41. Harry R, Auzinger G, Wendon J (2002) The clinical importance of adrenal insufficiency in acute hepatic dysfunction. Hepatology 36: 395-402
42. Auzinger G, Sizer E, Bernal W et al (2004) Incidence of lung injury in acute liver failure: diagnostic role of extravascular lung water index. Crit Care 8 (Suppl 1):40
43. Dellinger R.P, Levy MM, Carlet JM et al (2008) Surviving sepsis campaign: international Guidelines. Intensive Care Med 34:17-60
44. Donahoe M (2006) Basic ventilator management: lung protective strategies. Surg Clin North Am 6:1389-1408
45. Petrucci N, Iacovelli W (2007) Lung protective ventilation strategy for the acute respiratory distress syndrome. Cochrane Database of Systematic Reviews Issue 3, Art No CD003844
46. Lichtenstein DA, Mezieres GA 2008) Relevance of lung ultrasound in the diagnosis of acute respiratory failure: the BLUE protocol. Chest 134:117-125
47. Malbrain ML, Cheatham M (2004) Cardiovascular effects and optimal preload markers in intraabdominal hypertension. In: Vincent JL (ed) Yearbook of intensive care and emergency medicine, pp 519-543. Springer, New York
48. Moore K. Renal failure in ALF (1999) Eur J Gastroenterology 11:967-975
49. Hadengue A, Gadano A, Moreno R et al (1998) Beneficial effects of 2 day administration of terlipressin in patients with cirrhosis and hepatorenal syndrome. J Hepatology 29:565-570
50. Uriz J, Gines P, Cardenas A et al (2000) Terlipressin plus albumin infusion: an effective and safe therapy of hepatorenal syndrome. J Hepatology 33:43-48
51. Duvoux C, Zanditenas D, Hézode C et al (2002) Effects of noradrenalin and albumin in patients with type 1 hepatorenal syndrome: a pilot study. Hepatology 36:374-380

52. Ronco C, Bellomo R, Homel P et al (2000) Effects of different doses in continuous veno-venous haemofiltration on outcomes of acute renal failure: a prospective randomised trial. Lancet 356:1441

53. Mehta RL (2005) Continuous renal replacement therapy in the critically ill patient. Kidney Int 267:781-795

54. Fiaccadori E, Maggiore U, Rotelli C et al (2002) Continuous haemofiltration in acute renal failure with prostacyclin as the sole anti-haemostatic agent. Intensive Care Med28:586-593

55. Rolando N, Wade J, Davalos M et al (2000) The systemic inflammatory response syndrome in acute liver failure. Hepatology 232:734-739

56. Rolando N, Philpott-Howard J, Williams R (1996) Bacterial and fungal infection in acute liver failure. Semin Liver Dis 16:389-402

57. Vaquero J, Polson J, Chung C et al (2003) Infection and the progression of hepatic encephalopathy in acute liver failure. Gastroenterology 125:755-764

58. Antoniades CG, Berry PA, Davies ET et al (2006) Reduced monocyte HLA-DR expression: a novel biomarker of disease severity and outcome in acetaminophen induced acute liver failure. Hepatology 44:34-43

59. Rolando N, Gimson A, Wade J et al (1993) Prospective controlled trial of selective parenteral and enteral antimicrobial regimen in fulminant hepatic failure. Hepatology 17:196-201

60. Pittet D, Monod M, Suter PM et al (1994) Candida colonization and subsequent infections in critically ill surgical patients. Ann Surgery 220:751-758

61. De Jonge E, Schultz MJ, Spanjaard L et al (2003) Effects of selective decontamination of digestive tract on mortality and acquisition of resistant bacteria in intensive care: a randomised controlled trial. Lancet 362:1011- 1016

62. Koeman M, Van der Ven AJ, Hak E et al (2006) Oral decontamination with chlorhexidine reduces the incidence of ventilator-associated pneumonia. Am J Respir Crit Care Med 173:1348-1355

63. Pea F, Viale P, Furlanut M (2005) Antimicrobial therapy in critically ill patients. A review of pathophysiological conditions responsible for altered disposition and pharmacokinetic variability. Clin Parmacokinet 44:1009-1034

64. Pea F, Viale P, Pavan F, Furlanut M (2007) Pharmacokinetic considerations for antimicrobial therapy in patients receiving renal replacement therapy. Clin Pharmacokinet 46: 997-1038

65. Munoz SJ, Stravitz RT, Gabriel DA (2009) Coagulopathy of acute liver failure. Clin Liv Dis 13:95-107

66. Munoz S, Reddy KL, Lee W (2008) The coagulopathy of acute liver failure and implications for intracranial pressure monitoring. Neurocrit Care 9:103-107

67. De Gasperi, A. Corti, E. Mazza et al (2009) Acute liver failure: managing coagulopathy and the bleeding diathesis. Transpl Proc 41:1256-1259

68. De Gasperi A, Amici O, Mazza E et al (2006) Monitoring intraoperative coagulation. Transpl Proc 38:815-817

69. Singer AL, Olthoff KM, Haewon K et al (2001)A role of plasmapheresis in the management of acute hepatic failure in children. Ann Surg 234: 418-424

70. Shami V, Caldwell S, Hespenheide E (2003) Recombinant activated factor VII for the coagulopathy of fulminant hepatic failure compared with conventional therapy. Liver Transpl 9:138-143

71. Sembit S, Williams R. New liver support devices in ALF: a critical evaluation. Sem Liver Dis, 2003; 23: 283 – 294

72. Barshes NR, Gay AN, Williams B et al (2005) Support for the acutely failing liver: a comprehensive review of historic and contemporary strategies. J Am Coll Surg 201:458-476

73. Karvellas CJ, Gibney N, Kutsogiannis et al (2007) Bench-to-bedside review: Current evidence for extracorporeal albumin dialysis systems in liver failure. Crit Care 11:205

74. Liu JP, Gluud LL, Als-Nielsen B, Gluud C (2004) Artificial and bioartifcial support systems for liver failure. The Cochrane Database of Systematic Reviews, Issue 1, Art. No. CD003628 – Update 1 2009

75. McKanzie TJ, lillegard JB, Nyberg SL (2008) Artificial and bioartificial liver support. Semin liver Dis 28:210-217
76. Mintzner S, William R (2003) Albumin dialysis MARS 2003: what evidence, how to procede? Liver International 23:3-4
77. Lee KH, Lee MK H, Sutedja DS, Lim SG (2005) Outcome from MARS liver dialysis following drug induced liver failure. Liver International, 25: 973-977
78. Saliba F (2006) The MARS in the intensive care: a rescue therapy for patients with hepatic failure. Critical Care 10:118
79. Sauer IM, Goetz I, Walter G et al (2004) In vitro comparison of the MARS and SPAD. Hepatology 39:1408-1414
80. Rifai K, Ernst T, Kretschmer U et al (2003) Prometheus - a new extracorporeal system for the treatment of liver failure. J Hepatol 39:984-990
81. Ernst T, Kretschmer U, Hafer C et al (2005) The Prometheus device for extracorporeal support of combined liver and renal failure. Blood Purif 23:298
82. Demetriou A, Brown RS, Busuttil RW et al (2004) Prospective, randomized, multicenter, controlled trial of a Bioartificial Liver in treating acute liver failure. Ann Surg 239: 660-670
83. O'Grady J (2006) Personal view: current role of artificial liver support devices. Aliment Pharmacol Ther 23:1549-1557
84. Samuel D, Ichai P (2010) Prognosis indicator in acute liver failure: Is there a place for cell death markers? J Hepatol 53:593-595
85. Bechmann LP, Jochum C, Kocabayoglu P et al (2010) Cytokeratin 18-based modification of the Meld score improves prediction of spontaneous survival after acute liver failure. J Hepatol 53:639-647
86. Kramer DJ, Canabal JM, Arasi LC (2008) Application of intensive care medicine principles in the management of the acute liver failure patient. Liver Transplant 14:S85-S89
87. Larson AM. (2010) Diagnosis and management of acute liver failure. Current Opinion in Gastroenterology 26:214-221
88. Stravitz RT, Lefkowitch JH, Fontana RJ et al (2011) Autoimmune acute liver failure: Proposed clinical and histological criteria. Hepatology 53:517-526
89. De Backer D, Marx G, Tan A et al (2011) Arterial pressure-based cardiac output monitoring: a multicenter validation of the third-generation software in septic patients. Intensive Care Med 37:233-240
90. Monnet X, Lahner D (2011) Can the "FloTrac" really track flow in septic patients? Intensive Care Med 37:183-185
91. Stravits TR, Kramer DJ (2009) Management of acute liver failure. Nature Rev Gastroenterol Hepatol 6:542-513
92. Caironi P, Langer T, Taccone P et al (2010) Kidney instant monitoring (K.IN.G): a new analyzer to monitor kidney function. Minerva Anestesiol 76:316-324

Diuretics in Intensive Care: Positive and Negative Aspects

5

Pasquale Piccinni and Silvia Gramaticopolo

5.1 Introduction

Acute kidney injury is a frequent condition affecting critical patients. It is the clinician's responsibility to decide when it is best to initiate diuretic therapy and also which molecule to use and at what dosage. Such decision is based on a previous evaluation of the patient's volemic state and in consideration of the many difficulties that such an assessment presents when dealing with a critical patient. The clinician must finally be aware of the side effects of ongoing diuretic therapy in order to identify them and solve any related problem.

The liberal use of diuretics in intensive care patients is often justified by the need to maintain a non-oliguric state and also by the now obsolete concept of protecting the kidney from ischaemic damage. Diuretics are not linked to either reduced mortality or to increased frequency of renal replacement therapy (RRT). They are instead associated to less-prolonged RRT and to increased diuresis. There is a deep need for randomized controlled trials of critical patients with renal dysfunction.

Most of the studies involving the use of diuretics in this type of patient are retrospective and non-controlled. Shilliday [1] reports on the results of a randomized, double-blind, placebo-controlled prospective study which examines the effect of diuretics on renal function recovery, on the need for dialysis and on mortality and concludes that diuretic therapy promotes diuresis but it shows no evidence of also improving renal clearance. This confirms that the use of diuretics cannot be indiscriminate but must be selected on the basis of the patient's condition. The clinician must know every detail of diuretics pharmacokinetics and dynamics and recognize adverse events and interactions with other drugs. Each critical patient needs above all a clinician who can prescribe

P. Piccinni (✉)
Head of Anesthesiology and Resuscitation Department
Local Health Unit ULSS 6, Vicenza, Italy
e-mail: pasquale.piccinni@ulssvicenza.it

the most adequate treatment for his/her needs exactly at that particular moment of pathophysiological unbalance.

5.2   Epidemiology of Acute Renal Failure in the Critical Patient

Acute kidney injury (AKI) is characterized by the sudden decrease in glomerular filtrate rate (GFR) resulting in accumulation of urea and other toxins in the bloodstream.

The Acute Kidney Injury Network (AKIN), a panel of international interdisciplinary experts, has classified AKI according to RIFLE criteria (risk, injury, failure, loss and end-stage kidney disease) and has created a scale which reflects the progressively worsening levels of serum creatinine and of diuresis [2].

Acute kidney failure in critical patients is a high-impact daily occurrence in clinical practice. AKI incidence in intensive care varies from study to study depending on the patient population under treatment and on the level of importance of the referral centre (secondary or tertiary care); incidence is always higher in intensive care where there is a higher number of patients suffering from sepsis or multiple organ failure [3].

5.3   Pathophysiology of Critical Patients' Renal Function

The critical patient's kidney has in general a passive role and is victim to a precipitating event, often being totally unconnected to such event. In order to preserve renal function, measures must be taken to maintain optimal organ perfusion; nephrotoxic drugs should not be used and treatment must be planned in response to the primary pathological event. AKI patients very often suffer from fluid retention and volume overload which sometimes do not respond to diuretics administration.

Normal kidney function consists of three stages: glomerular filtration, fluid and solute reabsorption and urinary excretion. Diuretics act on the three processes and regulate volemia. Diuretics administration in the course of AKI has two objectives: kidney damage prevention and fluid overload management. A sustained diuresis eliminates sediment and avoids tubular obstruction as well as interstitial space reflux, the latter being the cause of renal damage [4].

It has also been suggested that loop diuretics lower renal tubule cells oxygen consumption thus protecting the kidney from ischaemic damage. Loop diuretics in fact inhibit the sodium-potassium-chloride pump which actively carries sodium (ATP consumption) [5]. Loop diuretics are frequently administered with a view to convert oliguric AKI into non-oliguric AKI and so improve prognosis; this treatment has however failed to provide any benefit to patients with acute tubular damage [5, 6].

According to available studies, the administration of diuretics in the early stages of AKI aims to facilitate fluid balance management, to contain electrolyte unbalance (hyperkalaemia, hypercalcaemia) but not to contain or prevent AKI progression.

5.4 Pharmacokinetics and Pharmacodynamics of Diuretics

IV diuretics are frequently employed in intensive care; they are essential in managing fluid balance. Several categories of diuretics are available: acetozolamide, spironolactone and potent loop diuretics. Loop diuretics are mostly used by intensive care doctors for patients with acute renal dysfunction. There is however little evidence that these drugs improve the outcome or have any protective action on renal failure.

Diuretics induce a loss of water and sodium; natriuretic drugs (peptides) induce a definite sodium loss, they promote glomerular filtration and inhibit sodium reabsorption; aquaretic drugs act on vasopressin 2 receptors (V_2R) in the renal collecting duct promoting excretion of solute-free water (aquaresis). Table 5.1 shows the various drugs and their respective site of action.

Diuretics are often administered in combination with vasoactive drugs that can modify cardiac output and vascular resistance and so increase renal perfusion, GFR and diuretics', aquaretics' and natriuretics' efficacy.

Several factors influence renal response: dosage, transport to site of action and bond with receptors. In severe multiple organ failure the drug response can be greatly altered by factors such as distribution volume and endothelial integrity or volemic overload, for instance, in a patient with heart failure.

5.4.1 Osmotic Diuretics: Mannitol

Mannitol is filtered by the glomerulus and is poorly reabsorbed by the renal tubule. It is relatively inert from a pharmacological point of view. Its sites of action are the loop of Henle and the proximal convoluted tubule and it draws solute-free water from the intracellular compartment. The effect of all osmotic diuretics is extra-cellular volume expansion, reduced blood viscosity and renin release inhibition; they increase renal blood flow and reduce medullary tonicity. With all these qualities, Mannitol has proved to be effective in reducing acute tubular necrosis damage in animal models but clinical application to patients has failed to produce sufficient proof. This drug's effect on humans is comparable, if not inferior, to abundant hydration [7, 8].

Table 5.1 Site and mechanism of action of drugs employed in volemia management

Group	Molecule	Drug example	Site of action	Renal Flow	IV Dose
Osmotic diuretics	Polisaccharide	Mannitol	PCT, loop of Henle	⇑⇑RBF, ⇑GFR	25-50 g
Carbon anhydrase inhibitors	Sulphonamide	Acetazolamide	PCT	⇓RBF, ⇓GFR	5 mg/kg
Loop diuretics	Sulphonamide	Furosemide	Loop of Henle ascending limb	⇑RBF, ⇔GFR	20-80 mg
DCT Diuretics	Benzothiadizine	Chlorothiazide	DCT	⇓RBF, ⇓GFR	0,5-1 g
K+ sparing diuretics	Steroid	Spironolactone	CD	⇔RBF, ⇔GFR	25-200 mg
DA agonists	Catecholamine	Dopamine	PCT	⇑⇑RBF, ⇔GFR	3-5 mg/kg/min
Natriuretic peptides	Peptide	Atrial natriuretic peptide	CD	⇑RBF, ⇔GFR	50 ng/kg/min
Vasopressin Antagonists (V2 receptors)	Amide	Conivaptan	CD	⇔RBF, ⇔GFR	20-40 mg

DA, Dopamine; *CD*, Collecting Duct; *GFR*, Glomerular Filtration Rate; *RBF*, Renal Blood Flow; *DCT*, Distal Convoluted Tubule; *PCT*, Proximal Convoluted Tubule.
Source: Mehta et al (2008) [24].

5.4.2 Loop Diuretics: Furosemide

Loop diuretics inhibit sodium-potassium-chloride pump of the apical membrane in the thick ascending limb of the loop of Henle. This process causes a general increase in Na^+, Cl^- and K^+ excretion and increased urine volume. Medullary osmotic gradient is reduced and so is free water reabsorption, regulated by antidiuretic hormone, in the collection tubules.

When administered orally, absorption varies between 65 and 100% but in current clinical practice furosemide continuous infusion is preferred to bolus injection given its greater efficacy and also with a view to avoid sudden fluctuations of intravascular volume [9]. Furosemide travels in the bloodstream after binding with albumin and albumin ensures that the drug arrives at the effector site; hypoalbuminemia significantly lowers the drug's efficacy.

Furosemide is potentially ototoxic as it may damage the organ of Corti.

5.4.3 Thiazides

Thiazide and thiazide-like diuretics are filtered by the nephron and excreted in the proximal tubule. They bind to Na^+ Cl^- cotransporter in the proximal part of the distal tubule. They promote potassium excretion through three mechanisms of action: increase in urine flow, increase of Na^+/K^+ exchange, increase in aldosterone release. Systemic effects are reduced extracellular volume, lower blood pressure through reduced cardiac output and also reduced glomerular filtrate. Pharmacokinetics criteria rely on one single oral dose and therefore exclude the use of this type of drug in a critical patient whose gastroenteric absorption is extremely variable and unpredictable.

5.4.4 Potassium-Sparing Diuretics

Spironolactone and its derivate, potassium canreonate, act as aldosterone antagonists. They block the aldosterone receptor from converting into active form thus inhibiting its effect. They bind to plasma proteins and are therefore dependent on such proteins for efficacious transport to the site of action. These drugs are usually administered in order to prevent hypokalaemia which is often induced by other diuretic drugs. The worst side effect is secondary hyperkalaemia which may sometimes develop. Due to the drugs' steroid structure, manifestations of androgen-like effects, or gynecomastia, or GI tract symptoms may appear.

5.4.5 Diuretic Peptides: Nesiritide

Nesiritide is the synthetic version of brain natriuretic peptide (BNP); its effects are vasodilation, natriuresis and diuresis.

Its use is endorsed by the fact that this drug shares the same characteristics of atrial natriuretic peptide (ANP); it increases GFR due to vasodilation of the afferent arteriole and to vasoconstriction of the efferent arteriole, it inhibits sodium re-uptake and redistributes blood flow in the medullary thus improving oxygen distribution and reducing its demand in the tubules. Despite these qualities, evidence does not support the use of natriuretic peptides in acute kidney failure but their use has been approved for acute decompensated heart failure.

Meta-analysis conducted to date on patients treated with nesiritide have shown a greater risk of renal failure and increased mortality at 30 days [10]. The use of nesiritide at very low dosage and in selected groups of patients after cardiac surgery is instead more promising.

5.4.6 Conivaptan

Vasopressin receptor antagonist drugs are, in theory, the ideal choice for the management of fluid overload in patients with heart failure. The FDA has approved the use of Conivaptan in the United States for the treatment of euvolemic or hypervolemic hyponaetremia.

Arginine vasopressin is the main regulator of free renal water reabsorption through vasopressin type2-receptors. The inhibition of this mechanism ensures a greater excretion of free water without depleting the system's sodium reserve [11].

5.4.7 Fenoldopam

Fenoldopam is a selectively active systemic vasodilator acting on dopamine type1-receptors. It inhibits proximal reabsorption of sodium and chloride and increases renal flow; it maintains or increases glomerular filtrate. It is the object of conjugation metabolism in the liver with no active metabolites. It is 88% bound to albumin and 90% excreted in the urine. Dose adjustment for hepatic or renal insufficiency is not required.

It is an extremely handy drug with a high safety profile. Several studies are taking place to evaluate its use for the prevention of renal injury in patients undergoing major cardiac or vascular surgery.

5.5 Diuretic Resistance Factors

The critical patient presents multiple diuretic resistance factors which have been examined mainly with regard to loop diuretics, i.e. furosemide. A pathophysiological consideration is that loop diuretics reduce circulating volume because of vasodilation mediated by prostaglandins, and increase diuresis; if the mechanism exceeds the expected result then the renal flow will decrease and consequently so will glomerular filtrate.

Pharmacologically sustained diuresis in a critical patient may suggest an adequate volemic state thus delaying intervention to maintain sufficient cardiac output. At the same time volemia prompts the activation of both adrenergic and renin-angiotensin systems giving rise to flow redistribution from renal cortex to medulla and so increasing sodium retention.

Besides pathophysiological considerations there are other factors which are clinically more evident: the presence of intratubular precipitates and hypoalbuminemia.

When there is tubule obstruction by Tamm-Horsfall proteins – and loop diuretics seem to also promote their aggregation – the diuretic drug may not reach its site of action, i.e. the sodium-potassium-chloride transporter in the ascending limb of the loop of Henle.

Hypoalbuminemia, typical for instance of nephrotic syndrome, increases the distribution volume of furosemide promoting its inactivation at extra-renal sites. Albumin is in fact furosemide main transporter to the tubular excretion site and albuminuria, due to furosemide bond with albumin, may limit the drug's efficacy at the effector site [4].

Pharmacodynamic and pharmacokinetic properties of any substance are sufficiently predictable under normal conditions but in the critical patient they vary to a great extent. Distribution volume may in such cases be normal, high or low and in any case extremely difficult to predict.

A no longer intact endothelium, a generalized inflammatory state, altered coagulation or simple fluid overload associated with cardiac failure make the treatment's efficacy quite unpredictable

5.6 Withdrawing Diuretic Treatment

Withdrawal of diuretic treatment should be considered in three cases:
1. when renal function is sufficient in maintaining euvolemia; renal function must then be evaluated on the basis of GFR and diuretics dosage must be adjusted accordingly. If diuresis increases while renal function improves, particular care must be placed on adequate volemia restoration in order to prevent hypotension episodes with the associated risk of ischaemia that would further damage renal tubules;
2. when there is no response to diuretic treatment. Loop diuretics should be avoided at the start of renal replacement therapy in order to limit the risk of ototoxicity;
3. when the risk of toxicity is high.

5.7   Diuretic Treatment in the Critical Patient

There is a lack of consensus on the use of diuretics in the presence of AKI despite their nearly routine administration in this context. Diuretics are contraindicated in hypovolemia but employed in the presence of euvolemia.

It is important that, initially, AKI be treated by fluid administration and vasoactive drugs [12] and that diuretic treatment be initiated only afterwards and once the patient's euvolemic state, without diuresis, has been restored.

When a patient presents clear signs of symptomatic fluid overload coupled with pulmonary oedema, loop diuretics are used in combination with other types of intervention aimed at optimizing haemodynamics.

A further indication for diuretic treatment is in fact the prevention of fluid overload in those patients undergoing abundant fluid administration therapy, i.e. patients suffering from acute lung injury (ALI), right or left insufficiency and lung transplant patients lacking lymphatic system. It is also common clinical practice to force diuresis in order to contain exogenous and endogenous intoxication (rhabdomyolysis etc.)

Several studies have been conducted in order to evaluate mortality incidence in intensive care patients treated with diuretics. We mention here the most relevant.

Mehta [13] has evaluated diuretic treatment influence on outcome in 552 renal failure patients who underwent nephrology consultation in intensive care at four university hospitals. Diuretics were already in use for 59% of the admitted patients prior to being examined and 12% of the patients underwent diuretic treatment the following week. The authors reported a higher risk of both hospital mortality and failed renal function recovery in the patient group that had been treated with diuretics. It is obviously noted that patients with severe liver failure probably require a greater degree of diuretic therapy and are therefore subject to higher mortality risk.

In a study conducted under the BEST Kidney (Beginning and Ending Supportive Therapy for the Kidney) initiative, 1,743 intensive care patients undergoing RRT or presenting severe renal failure were prospectively recruited and monitored up until discharge or death. Three different models of multivariate analysis were employed to test the link between diuretics use and mortality. No difference was found between patients receiving diuretics and patients not treated and it was concluded that diuretics administration in acute renal failure patients does not carry the risk of higher mortality [14].

Other randomized and controlled clinical studies aiming to evaluate loop diuretics effect on patients suffering from confirmed AKI have revealed increased diuresis without any change in clinical outcome such as mortality, renal function recovery or need for dialysis [1, 15, 16].

A recent retrospective analysis by Bagshaw where the results of 62 studies were reviewed has concluded that the use of loop diuretics is not associated with either lower mortality or independence from RRT [17].

Clinical studies confirm that diuretics increase diuresis but fail to prove that they are truly beneficial to the renal function.

5.8 Prophylactic Administration of Diuretics for the Prevention of AKI and of Radiocontrast-Induced Nephropathy

The mechanism of action of loop diuretics in particular [18] could suggest that furosemide might prevent AKI since it lowers medullary oxygen consumption and prevents renal tubule obstruction and filtrate reflux by promoting urinary flow. Only a few and contradictory facts however support the use of diuretics for such purpose.

Contrast injection is the most frequent cause of acute changes in the renal function but its pathogenesis has yet to be fully clarified.

Many studies prove that sole volemic expansion compared to furosemide-induced expansion results in the same creatinine increase for both groups and in fact the increase is higher for the group treated also with furosemide [7, 19, 20, 21].

A recent retrospective analysis of 41 randomized trials has underlined how furosemide, dopamine and mannitol increase the risk of contrast-induced nephropathy [22].

A study conducted on patients who had undergone major surgery has not shown any improvement in creatinine clearance in the patients treated with a low dose of furosemide following surgery [23].

5.9 The Patient with Acutization of Chronic Renal Failure

A patient with chronic renal failure who also experiences acute renal injury is often resistant to diuretic therapy. There is a global reduction of sodium reabsorption and a counter increase of K and Cl absorption. Sodium reabsorption is however relatively higher at distal tubule level as a natural counterbalancing occurrence and this can in some cases assist the clinician in boosting diuresis.

A natural resistance to diuretic therapy is often present in chronic renal failure and this is due to several factors:
• it is more difficult for the diuretic drug to reach the effector site;
• acidosis due to organic anions increase and urea accumulation limit the drug's efficacy.

It is sometimes useful to combine a loop diuretic with thiazide which acts on the distal tubule tract and prevents reabsorption of sodium, chloride and water. This combination promotes fluid excretion but cannot cause hypokalaemia or further increase of creatinine.

For patients with a chronic renal condition and an initial resistance to diuretic therapy it would seem useful, at times, to combine furosemide with an

ACE-inhibitor (ACE-I), a sartan drug, a calcium-antagonist drug. Potassium-sparing diuretics must obviously be avoided. Nephrologists nonetheless share the opinion that such combinations should be avoided and that, if treatment is already in place, it should be withdrawn. It is their belief that ACE-I and/or sartan drugs could result in functional deterioration due to altered haemodinamics. It is also imperative to mention that calcium-antagonist drugs tend to promote sodium retention [24].

5.10   Diuretic Treatment in Cardiac Failure

Acute cardiac decompensation requires diuretic treatment to limit the patient's volemic overload. There are no detailed guidelines on a preferred class of diuretics. Thiazide-like diuretics are administered when a strong hypotensive action is necessary; spironolactone appears to increase survival and it is therefore administered to patients with serum creatinine not above 2 or 2.5mg/dL [25].

The treatment of acute cardiac decompensation has lately acquired a further tool: nesiritide, a synthetic BNP analogue, which in combination with the "classical" treatment for decompensation has proved to be effective in reducing pulmonary capillary pressure and in resolving dyspnea [26]. Other studies have however shown increased creatinine levels and lack of natriuretic effect [10].

Acute renal failure is a frequent complication in cardiac surgery patients. Prophylactic administration of furosemide, in this context, proved to be no better than a placebo and also proved to be linked to a relative increase of creatinine in the patients treated [27].

Nesiritide increases renal perfusion flow and glomerular filtration at the same time inhibiting aldosterone release. The NAPA trial proved that continuous infusion of nesiritide at a low dose of 0.01 µg/kg/min and extracorporeal support in patients with left ventricular failure who underwent aortocoronary bypass surgery produced an improvement of post-surgical function and possibly increased survival [28].

The studies conducted with nesiritide have been just as encouraging and have proven the drug to be effective at very low dose continuous infusion of 0.005 µg/kg/min when administered to patients with diminished renal function who underwent cardiac surgery. There was a decrease of plasma cystatin, the most sensitive marker of renal function, and aldosterone release was inhibited. [29].

The use of different molecules, such as fenoldopam (dopamine-1-receptor agonist) and adenosine A1-receptor antagonists have been evaluated for treating resistance to diuretic therapy but, to date, the results have not been conclusive [24].

The early start of renal replacement therapy to reduce volume overload is of the utmost importance in patients suffering from cardiac failure and not responding adequately to diuretic treatment.

5.11   Diuretic Treatment in Respiratory Failure

The FACTT study conducted within the ARDS Clinical Trials Network has compared 1000 ALI patients treated by restricted fluid administration and by free fluid administration. The target for the group conservatively treated was PVC < 4 mm/Hg or PAOP (pulmonary artery occlusion pressure) < 8 mm/Hg. For the group liberally treated the targets were PVC 10-14 mm/Hg and PAOP 14-18 mm/Hg.

The study revealed a similar 60-day-mortality rate for both groups but the patients conservatively treated benefitted from better respiratory exchange and from a shorter time on mechanical ventilation and in the intensive care unit. These patients also presented a negative fluid balance for a higher number of days, a greater serum oncotic pressure, slightly higher creatininaemia and BUN and they required increased use of furosemide. The number of days clear of renal failure and need for RRT were however similar for both groups [30].

These facts suggest that the ALI patient should receive loop diuretics so that a lower fluid balance is maintained and extrapulmonary water is reduced whilst considering that renal function indicators may become moderately altered without serious consequences.

5.12   Diuretic Treatment in Liver Failure

The patient with portal hypertension presents increased nitric oxide level resulting in vasodilation and relative arterial hypovolemia which in turn stimulates the renin-angiotensin-aldosterone system. A condition of splanchnic vasodilation, hypotension and renal hypoperfusion arises with associated vasopressin release and decrease in free water excretion.

Ascites treatment requires sodium intake restriction and combined therapy with furosemide and spironolactone. Paracentesis must be carried out for serious ascites and when the fluid consists of more than 5 L it must be combined with albumin or colloid administration to prevent high risk of hepatorenal syndrome.

Hepatorenal syndrome is a form of acute renal failure due to a significant reduction of systemic defences resulting in compensatory renal vasoconstriction. In order to maintain renal perfusion, the treatment is targeted at reducing splanchnic vasodilation by means of vasopressin V1-receptor agonist agents. Ornipressin and terlipressin have been used in the course of some interesting trials. Both drugs act mainly on splanchnic circulation. Terlipressin in combination with albumin has produced the best results. The vasoconstrictor effect is linked to ischaemic complications. Other studies sharing the same pursuit have been conducted on alpha-receptors agonists such as noradrenaline and the results have been equally promising [24, 31].

5.13 Diuretic Treatment in Sepsis

Acute liver failure is a very common complication of sepsis. Volemia restoration by infusion of fluids with a view to optimizing oxygen transport is the main priority in a septic patient. A deduction based on pathophysiology could be that optimized volemia also ensures optimized renal perfusion but it lacks verification.

With regard to the type of fluids employed in resuscitating a septic patient, the studies so far conducted have often not been aimed at evaluating such fluids' impact on the renal function but it is possible to gather some information from the available data. The use of gels and colloid solutions, when compared to the use of sole crystalloid solutions, appears to be an independent factor with regard to renal damage in the presence of sepsis. These data have been confirmed by a study on transplanted kidneys where cytological damage by osmosis had been observed in those patients who had been treated with colloid solution (hydroxyethyl starch) [32]. The use of hypertonic saline solution seems instead more promising; some studies reveal how this solution temporarily improves haemodynamics and oxygen transport besides having an anti-inflammatory effect. The impact of hypertonic saline solution on renal failure and on the need for RRT has not yet been verified [33]. The study on Early Goal-Directed Therapy by E.P. Rivers reveals that an early and aggressive infusion therapy in a septic patient optimizes systemic circulation and in turn also the renal flow. There are however no studies for the investigation of outcome in relation to the kidney following this approach [34]. It is obvious that once systemic perfusion has been optimized and an adequate cardiac output has been reached but diuresis remains unsatisfactory, further fluid administration would probably be ineffective in sustaining renal blood flow; it would instead contribute to a positive fluid balance, a damaging event for patients suffering from acute pulmonary damage.

Current guidelines for sepsis treatment favour early intervention with RRT, as soon as the onset of diuretic therapy-resistant oliguria is evident. RRT may be continuous or intermittent depending on the patient's haemodynamic condition [35].

5.14 Conclusion

The critical patient in intensive care is actually exposed to greater AKI risk factors and is also subject to fluid overload by infusion therapy, vasopressors and nutritional support.

The use of diuretics in these patients must be targeted to volemia optimization rather than to AKI prevention or containment. The indication for diuretic therapy is fluid overload management and not oliguria treatment.

It is important to determine and optimize the critical patient's volemic state, a process which requires the administration of diuretics to ensure transition to non-oliguric AKI; these conditions allow for an easier management of the intensive care patient.

Bibliography

1. Shilliday IR, Quinn KJ, Allison MEM (1997) Loop diuretics in the management of acute renal failure: a prospective, double-blind, placebo-controlled, randomized study. Nephrology Dialysis Transplantation 12:2592-2596
2. Mehta RL, Kellum JL, Shah SV et al (2007) Acute Kidney Injury Network: report of an initiative to improve outcomes in acute kidney injury. Crit Care 11:R31
3. Cruz DN, Ronco C (2007) Acute kidney injury in the intensive care unit: current trends in incidence and outcome. Critical Care 11:149
4. Karajala V, Mansour W, Kellum JA (2009) Diuretics in acute kidney injury. Minerva Anestesiologica 75:251-257
5. Brezis M, Rosen S, Silva P et al (1984) Transport activity modifies thick ascending limb damage in the isolated perfused kidney. Kidney Int 25: 65-72
6. Kellum JA, Bellomo R, Ronco C (2007) The concept of acute kidney injury and the RIFLE criteria. Contirb Nephrol 156:10-16
7. Solomon R, Werner C, Mann D et al (1994) Effects of saline, mannitol and furosemide to prevent acute decreases in renal function induced by radiocontrast agents. N Engl J Med 331:1416-1420
8. Homsi E, Barreiro MF, Orlando JM et al (1997) Prophylaxis of acute renal failure in patients with rhabdomyolysis. Ren Fail 19:283-288
9. Salvador DR, Rey NR, Ramos GC et al (2005) Continuous infusion versus bolus injection of loop diuretics in congestive heart failure. Cochrane Database Syst Rev CD003178
10. Sackner-Bernstein JD, Kowalski M, Fox M et al (2005) Short-term risk of death after treatment with nesiritide for decompensated heart failure: a pooled analysis of randomized controlled trials. JAMA 293:1900-1905
11. Yukinori A, Fujimori A, Sasamata M et al (2009) New topics in vasopressin receptors and approach to novel drugs: research and development of Conivaptan Hydrochloride (YM087), a drug for the treatment of hyponatremia. J Pharmacol Sci 109:53-59
12. Pinsky MR, Brophy P, Padilla J et al (2008) Fluid and volume monitoring. Int J Artif Organs31:111-126
13. Mehta Rl, Pascual Mt, Soroko S et al (2002) Diuretics, mortality, and nonrecovery of renal function in acute renal failure. JAMA 288: 2547-2553
14. Uchino S, Doig GS, Bellomo R et al (2004) Diuretics and mortality in acute renal failure. Crit Care Med 32:1669-1677
15. Shilliday I, Allison ME (1994) Diuretics in acute renal failure. Ren Fail 16:3-17
16. Cantarovich F, Rangoonwala B, Lorenz H et al (2004) High-dose furosemide for established ARF: a prospective, randomized, double-blind, placebo-controlled, multicenter trial. Am J Kidney Dis 44: 402-409
17. Bagshaw SM, Delaney A, Haase M et al (2007) Loop diuretics in the management of acute renal failure: a systematic review and meta-analysis. Crit Care Resusc 9:60-68
18. Schetz M (2004) Should we use diuretics in acute renal failure? Best Prac Res Clin Anaesthesiol 18:75-89
19. Dussol B, Morange S, Loundoun A et al (2006) A randomized trial of saline hydration to prevent contrast nephropathy in chronic renal failure patients. Nephrol Dial Transplant 21:2120-2126
20. Stevens MA, Mccullough PA, Tobin KJ et al (1999) A prospective randomized trial of prevention measures in patients at high risk for contrast nephropathy: results of the PRINCE Study (Prevention of Radiocontrast Induced Nephropathy Clinical Evaluation) J Am Coll Cardiol 33:403-411

21. Weinstein JM, Heyman S, Brezis M (1992) Potential deleterious effect of furosemide in radiocontrast nephropathy. Nephron 62:413-415
22. Kelly AM, Dwamena B, Cronin P et al (2008) Meta-analysis: effectiveness of drugs for preventing contrast-induced nephropathy. Ann Intern Med 148:284-294
23. Hager B, Betschart M, Krapf R (1996) Effect of postoperative intravenous loop diuretic on renal function after major surgery. Schweiz Med Wochenschr 126:666-673
24. Mehta RL, Cantarovich F, Shaw A et al (2008) Pharmacologic approaches for volume excess in acute kidney injury (AKI). Int J Artif Organs31:127-144
25. Hunt SA et al (2005) ACC/AHA 2005 guideline update for the diagnosis and management of chronic heart failure in the adult- summary article: A report of the American College of Cardiology/ American Heart Association Task Force on Practice Guidelines (Writing Committee to update the 2001 guidelines for the evaluation and management of heart failure). J Am Coll Cardiol 46:1116-1143
26. Colucci WS, Elkayam U, Horton DP et al (2000) Intravenous nesiritide, a natriuretic peptide, in the treatment of decompensated congestive heart failure. Nesiritide Study Group. N Engl J Med 343:246-253
27. Lassnigg A, Donner E, Grubhofer G et al (2000) Lack of renoprotective effects of dopamine and furosemide during cardiac surgery. J Am Soc Nephro 11:97-104
28. Mentzer RM Jr, Oz MC, Sladen RN et al (2007) Effects of perioperative nesiritide in patients with left ventricular dysfunction undergoing cardiac surgery: the NAPA Trial. J Am Coll Cardiol 49:716-726
29. Horng HC, Thoralf MS, David JC et al (2007) Low dose nesiritide and the preservation of renal function in patients with renal dysfunction undergoing cardiopulmonary-bypass surgery. A double-blind placebo-controlled pilot study. Circulation 116 (Suppl I)134-138
30. ARDS Clinical Trials Network (2006) Comparison of two fluid-management strategies in acute lung injury. N Engl J Med 354:2564-2575
31. Alessandria C, Ottobrelli A, Debernardi-Venon W et al (2007) Noradrenalin vs terlipressin in patients with hepatorenal syndrome: a prospective, randomized, unblinded, pilot study. J Hepatol 47:499-505
32. Citanova ML, Mavre J, Riou B et al (2001) Long-term follow-up of transplanted kidneys according to plasma volume expander of kidney donors. Inten Care Med 27:1830
33. Bagshaw SM, Bellomo R (2006) Fluid resuscitation and the septic kidney. Curr Opin Crit Care 12:527-530
34. Rivers E, Nguyen B, Havstad S et al (2001) Early goal-directed therapy in the treatment of severe sepsis and septic shock. N Engl J Med 345:1368-1377
35. Dellinger PR, Levy MM, Carlet MJ (2008) Surviving Sepsis Campaign: International guidelines for management of severe sepsis and septic shock - 2008. Crit Care Med 36:296-327

Perioperative and Intensive Care Management of Haemorrhage: the Opinion of the Haemathologist

6

Marco Marietta

6.1 Introduction

Why address haemorrhage and why do we need the haemathologist's opinion? The reason is that today massive haemorrhage is still a relevant clinical problem in a number of different situations. Uncontrollable haemorrhage accounts for 40% of trauma deaths, 60% of which occur after hospital admission [1-5] but it can also affect major surgery procedures such as organ transplant, cardiac and hepatic surgery increasing their mortality rate by up to 20% [6, 7].

Such great clinical importance is met by relatively scant scientific knowledge starting with the nosographic definition of haemorrhage. Massive haemorrhage may in fact be defined according to a scale of different events [8, 9]:
- loss of total blood volume within 24 hours;
- loss of 50% of blood volume within 3 hours;
- loss of blood at a rate of 150 mL/min;
- loss of blood at a rate of 1.5 mL/kg/min for 20 min or longer.

The notion of massive haemorrhage is associated to massive transfusion, which consists of total blood volume replacement within 24 hours [8-10]. This is equivalent to 7% of the ideal body weight of an adult and to 8-9% in a child or to 10 blood units (PRC) in a 70 kg male.

It is clearly difficult, if not impossible, to validate the effectiveness and the safety of treatments according to Evidence Based Medicine methods in the presence of such complex and varied pathology that even lacks a univocal definition. The treatment of critical bleeding continues to be largely empirical and poorly codified.

M. Marietta (✉)
Department of Oncology and Haematology
University of Modena and Reggio Emilia, Modena, Italy
e-mail: marco.marietta@unimore.it

Biagio Allaria (ed.), *Practical Issues in Anesthesia and Intensive Care*
© Springer-Verlag Italia 2012

Under the circumstances the only possible approach is to start from the pathophysiology of haemorrhage and in particular from the extraordinary in vivo models made up of congenital bleeding disorders attributable to individual flaws of coagulation factors. The complete picture can be obtained from this starting point and the haematologist may provide useful insight into this difficult task.

6.2   Haemostasis Overview (or "Haemostasis for Dummies")

The recurring nightmare of medical students and of many doctors is undoubtedly represented by the "coagulation cascade", an excellent example of how mnemonic learning of an abstract concept is destined to failure. Haemostasis is in fact very simple and it is possible to identify its own logic by reproducing the coagulation process through the use of simple geometric shapes [11].

The logic of haemostasis consists in the amplification and localisation of coagulation reactions. Line, point and triangle are sufficient to represent the concept in graphic form (Fig. 6.1). The line represents the undamaged endothelium, a normally non-thrombogenic surface; the point is where the endothelium loses its anatomical or functional integrity and precipitates a series of reactions (the cascade) that in turn amplify the alarm signal.

It is evident that the triggering of these reactions to physiological conditions is located on the sub-endothelial surface, so as to immediately raise the alarm that an interruption is taking place in the endothelium that is normally undamaged and working. The process that leads to clot formation must however remain in place on the lesion site, hence the triangle shape, and to this end inhibitor signals initiate in the undamaged endothelium (Fig. 6.2).

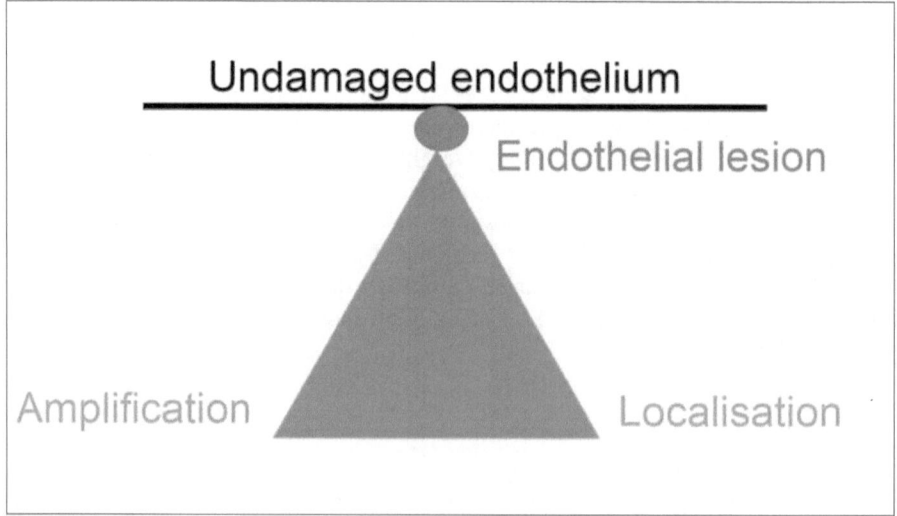

Fig. 6.1 Schematic representation of haemostasis

Fig. 6.3 shows a graphic synthesis of the processes leading to the activation of the plasma phase of coagulation. The activation signal relies on the ability of tissue factor, a sub-endothelial transmembrane molecule, to bind with activated Factor VII, a minimal quantity of which is present in the blood, and to trigger both the further activation of Factor VII and the activation of Factor X [12]. Factor X with cofactor V can convert prothrombin to thrombin, and thrombin is the real key to coagulation since not only does it convert soluble fibrinogen into insoluble fibrin, but also it further amplifies the signal both at plasma and platelet levels [11, 12].

- Amplification
- Quick initial response (continuous minimal activation)
- Localisation
- Activation mechanisms (normally in subendothelium)
- Inhibition mechanisms (normally on endothelium)

Fig. 6.2 The rationale of haemostasis

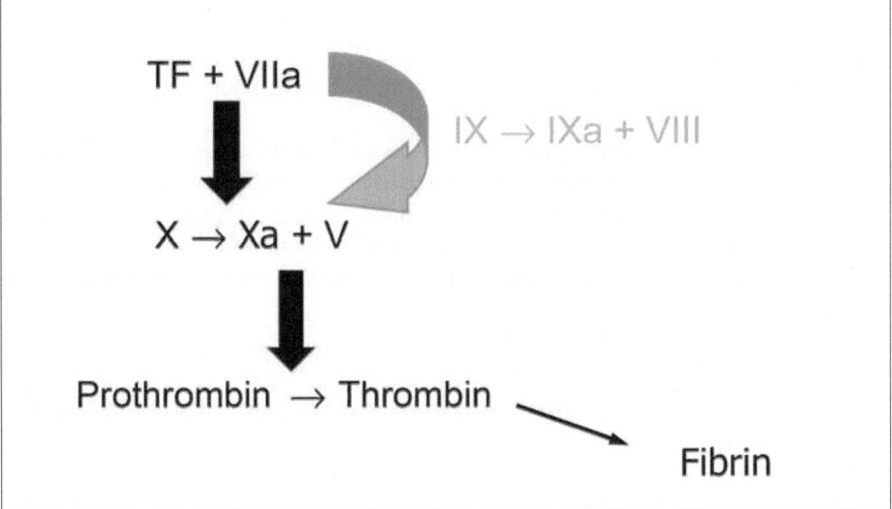

Fig. 6.3 The coagulation cascade

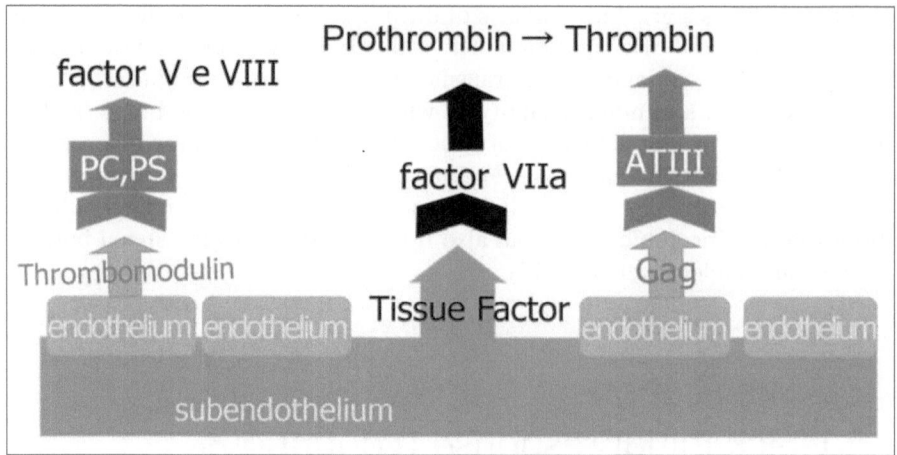

Fig. 6.4 Localisation of signals for coagulation activation and inhibition

In physiological haemostasis this process is the first line of defence, as it is readily available and relied upon to provide a first dose of thrombin in a short period of time; the same process is just as readily controlled by the tissue factor pathway inhibitor (TFPI). If the stimulus for the activation of haemostasis is constant, then a parallel, albeit slower, process is delegated to provide a continuous supply of thrombin. In this parallel process the TF/VIIa complex activates Factor IX and subsequent interaction of Factor IX and VIII activates Factor X and the final common pathway:

- the interaction of Factor VIIa and TF starts coagulation;
- the newly-formed complex activates the next phases in two ways:
  - by activating Factor IX which interacts with Factor VIII and the resulting complex in turn activates Factor X;
  - by directly activating Factor X;
- Factor X, however activated, forms a complex with Factor V and converts prothrombin (II) to thrombin.

Another important element is haemostasis process localisation. This is evident if we take into consideration the pathological conditions of its absence, such as thrombosis and disseminated intravascular coagulation, and it is made possible by the presence of the healthy endothelium upstream and downstream of the lesion, where the coagulation standard inhibitors are expressed (Fig. 6.4).

6.3   Haemostatic System and Haemostasis: the Trauma Model

A poly-trauma and massively bleeding patient forces us to take a new and holistic approach to physiological haemostasis. The most frequently observed haemostatic system failures relate to conditions where only one of this complex framework is altered: typical examples are congenital coagulation disorders such as haemophilia and coagulation factors deficiency, or thrombocytopenia. In such conditions, it has been noted that an adequate haemostasis can be ensured by providing very low levels of the missing element: approximately 10% of the factors physiological values and 10,000 platelets/mmc is sufficient. This is not surprising, since if you take into account the key role of the haemostatic system in ensuring the survival of the individual, it is easy to conclude that it has developed with a great degree of redundancy. Such system redundancy can be better comprehended by analyzing a totally different in vivo model, namely the polytrauma coagulopathy [3, 5, 13, 14]. In this complex and serious pathology, the whole haemostatic system is adversely impacted by a variety of known elements, detailed below (Fig. 6.5).

1. *Coagulation by dilution*: massive haemodilution is caused by high-volume infusion of crystalloids and colloids and involves a reduction of coagulation factors levels and platelet count. Employing a high molecular weight hydroxyethyl starch (HES) may result in a marked reduction of the FVIII-von Willebrand levels, causing an acquired von Willebrand syndrome and a coagulation disorder, which is however corrected by the infusion of fibrinogen [15]. Additionally, it has been noted that saline hypertonic solutions (although easily administered in emergency situations) have a negative effect, altering both the haemostatic tests and the platelet functionality [16, 17].

2. *Acidosis*: acidosis results from a reduced perfusion and anaerobic metabolism due to lactic acid build up; even a negligible pH variation compromises both the function of coagulation enzymes and platelets. A mere pH value reduction from 7.4 to 7 decreases prothrombin activation by the prothrombin complex (Xa/FVa) by 70% [3, 18]. This is due to several fac-

- Dilutional coagulopathy
- Hypothermia
- Acidosis
- Anaemia
- Hyperfibrinolysis

Fig. 6.5 Trauma coagulopathy

tors, related both to the haemocoagulation phase (enzyme malfunction, incorrect binding to Ca++, hypofibrinogenaemia by sequestration and degradation) and to the platelet activation phase (50% reduction in the platelet count and structural variation). An aspect promoting acidosis relates to the bags of concentrated erythrocytes used for transfusion with approximately 30% of the bags being stored for over 3 weeks: in that time, the concentrated erythrocytes Base Excess jumps from −20 mmol/L to −50 mmol/L [19]. It follows that massive transfusion of "old" bags of erythrocytes could be regarded as a contributing factor to the aggravation of acidosis already present due to aerobic metabolism changes secondary to trauma. Acidosis may be corrected either by sodium bicarbonate (NaHCO3) or by tri-hydroxymethyl-aminomethane (THAM), but the respective results on the haemostatic system appear to be different; some data indicate that whilst both can reduce pH and Base Excess values, the former is unable to improve thrombin production whereas THAM, in animal models, is associated with stabilizing thrombin production at normal levels [20, 21].

3. *Hypothermia*: slows down the coagulation cascade enzyme process, modifies the fibrinolytic system balance by increasing deficit of typical system inhibitors (e.g. PAI and alpha-2-antiplasmin), and reduces platelet function. Reduced production of Tromboxane B2 (a platelet activation indicator) has been observed, as well as lower platelet aggregation, attributable to the failed expression of GMP-140 and of the GPIb-IX complex. The consequences of hypothermia-induced coagulopathy are severe; it has been shown that at a temperature of < 33°C the activity of an otherwise healthy haemostatic system is reduced by an amount comparable to that of a normothermic system with factor levels < 50% [22]. Additionally, hypothermia and acidosis have a synergic effect on coagulopathy [23], a very significant consideration from the clinical point of view, in that the two conditions are almost without exception to be found in a patient suffering from massive haemorrhage. A recent study [24] has analysed through a TEG (Thromboelastography) of an animal model the pathophysiologic mechanism of hypothermia-induced coagulopathy and the results show that hypothermia causes both a platelet disorder and an abnormally low platelet count, whilst dilution coagulopathy is associated to a reduced clot consistency, in turn due to hypofibrinogenaemia.

4. *Anaemia*: tests have shown that a 20% haematocrit can inhibit platelet adhesion and aggregation in a manner similar to that observed with platelet values as low as 20,000/mmc: this is because the number and size of red blood cells, as indicated by the Ht value, are the components that determine platelets radial movement and their adhesion to sub-endothelial activation signals [25]. In regular flow conditions, platelet adhesion rate increases five fold when the Ht value increases from 10% to 40%, but no further change is noted above a 40% increase, indicating the saturation of the transport capability of the red blood cells. Such saturation, however, is

not observed where the platelet adhesion mechanism is prevalent, as in the presence of widespread endothelial damage. In this latter condition the platelet adhesion and the clot formation rates show a linear increase in line with the Ht value increase from 10% up to 70% [26]. From pathophysiologic data stems the clinical consideration that Ht optimum value, with regard to haemostasis, is higher than that required for standard oxygenation. This does not necessarily imply that the current transfusion procedures should be revised upwards since such choice should take into account many more factors, including significant organisation and management considerations. It is however important for the intensivist to bear the pathophysiologic data in mind in order to optimise transfusional treatment of haemorrhagic patients, taking also into account the option to reach and maintain Ht values of 30% [14, 27], as suggested by some of the authors.

5. *Hyperfibrinolysis*: studying this vital phase of haemostasis is a difficult process; for this reason our knowledge of the role it plays in the patient's coagulopathy is somewhat limited. The data on fibrinolytic system response to the onset of haemorrhage are contradictory: in the case of tissue damage both tPA and PAI values increase, whilst in a severe trauma tPA value increase is higher than PAI Type 1 value, resulting in hyperfibrinolysis and in consumption of coagulation factors. A recent study utilising TEG has shown the presence of hyperfibrinolysis in 6% of trauma patients, which also proves the correlation of data, severity of the trauma and outcome [28].

6. *Hypocalcaemia*: low plasma levels of ionized calcium are often found in seriously ill patients and are associated to a higher mortality rate (hazard ratio = 5.1 for < 0.90 mmol/L and 1.8 for values between 0.90 and 1.15 mmol/L) [29]. Hypocalcaemia can be made worse by the infusion of citrate present in transfused haemocomponents. The few data available regarding the dosage-response effect of hypocalcaemia on haemostasis indicate that thrombin production is reduced only when ionized calcaemia values are lower than 0.6-0.7 mmol/L [30]. It should however be noted that with calcaemia values lower than 0.8-0.9 mmol/L cardiac problems requiring emergency intervention are very frequent and therefore in medical practice the related haemostatic problems are seldom observed, since any deficit of this ion is rectified before it is detected during the coagulation process.

The above pathophysiologic notions have a considerable clinical impact primarily by reminding us of the necessity to optimise the "non-haemostatic" treatment of patients with poly-trauma haemorrhage (adjusting hypothermia and acidosis, optimising crystalloids and colloids use to restore volemia.) A second and just as important consideration concerns the "minimum" values of each component likely to achieve a satisfactory haemostasis. It is clear that when such significant changes occur in various points of the system, the thresholds previously quoted (10% of each factor, 10,000 platelets) will no longer be sufficient to ensure an adequate outcome and it would be advisable to adopt a much more aggressive remedial procedure which will restore as much as possible of the functionality of the haemostatic system as a whole.

6.4   Laboratory Monitoring of Massive Haemorrhage

Most of the guidelines relating to the treatment of massive haemorrhage [31-33] emphasise that types and quantities of the haemoderivatives used to replace the lost volumes should be determined on the basis of laboratory tests. It is appreciated that it is essential to start the treatment with fresh plasma when the volume transfused to the patient is equal to or higher than one blood volume (an indicative quantity is 70 mL/kg) and when haemostasis tests are not readily available; this is because it has been noted that replacing one blood volume with a concentrate of erythrocytes and crystalloids and colloids implies a reduction in the coagulation factors to 30% of the standard value, which could precipitate the onset of coagulopathy [34].

In practice, the emergency routine haemostasis tests available are of little use firstly because although the time required to carry them out is relatively short, any information provided is soon superseded by the rapidly changing overall clinical picture. To overcome this problem, analytical *point-of-care* systems have been developed and validated and they have proved to be quick and reliable, although it must be said that some issues remain in respect of the correlation to the standard coagulations tests, particularly APTT [35].

But it is not simply a matter of time. It is also an epistemological issue, in that the standard haemostatic tests provide a snap-shot of a complex and ever changing system and do not investigate the complexity of the system as a whole. Additionally, the tests totally overlook some of the system phases that are of critical clinical importance (such as fibrinolysis).

Thromboelastography [TEG] appears to be the only answer to the need for a comprehensive and quick test that may be carried out at the patient's bedside even by unskilled medical personnel [36, 37]. Numerous studies have endorsed such a method and have demonstrated that it would assist in identifying the early stages of haemostasis failure in trauma patients [38] and in investigating the fibrinolysis issues [28, 39]. Additionally, it has come to light that the predictability delivered by the TEG test of the need for a transfusion is higher than that delivered by traditional haemostatic tests (PT, APTT) [40] and is therefore used as a routine method in many centres as a means to address the transfusion strategies for trauma patients – a practice already adopted in cardiac surgery [41].

It is important for all this information to translate into a sensible and cautious approach on the part of the clinical staff. Having stated that the TEG test is a useful tool to manage these patients, it should be noted that there are a number of associated issues to be fully investigated, first of all the standardisation issue and therefore it must not take the place of an accurate clinical evaluation in the broad sense.

6.5   Treatment of Massive Haemorrhage

The treatment of massive haemorrhage comprises three basic stages:
- identification of the source;
- tissue oxygenation;
- haemostasis.

We will briefly review the first two stages, since they concern primarily intensive care treatment, and we will discuss in greater detail the third stage, which is more closely related to haematology.

6.5.1   Identification of the Source

Identifying the source of the haemorrhage, difficult though it may be at times, is the first, the most important and intuitive way of controlling the problem [42]. The process may require surgery, employing so called *damage control surgery* that may involve resuscitative thoracotomy and/or emergency laparotomy; this may be deemed necessary when haemorrhagic shock occurs both in the event of an abdominal crush trauma, associated to the presence of excess fluid in the abdomen, and in the event of a penetrating trauma [42, 43]. Interventional radiology, too, is taking an ever increasing active role in the management of such patients because it provides the opportunity to perform both embolisation of the affected blood vessels and cauterisation of haemorrhagic foci which would be otherwise difficult to access through thermal and mechanical action of high-intensity ultrasounds [42, 43]. A potentially important role is apparently assigned to a variety of local haemostatic compounds, which act by inducing a higher concentration and a local activation of coagulation factors [44]. These products have proved effective both in animal experimental models and in actual war scenarios; however, it must be said that their effectiveness and safety in massive poly-trauma and post-surgical haemorrhage situations has yet to be validated in precisely targeted trials [42, 44].

6.5.2   Tissue Oxygenation

Maintaining adequate tissue oxygenation during the initial treatment of trauma patients is a vital as much as an obvious goal. Although this has been the subject of many studies and reports, controversy still rages over the most effective transfusion strategy advice, possibly due to the absence of randomized controlled trials that put side by side and compare various transfusion strategies.

From the data available, it appears that a correlation exists between volume of transfused haemoderivatives and worse outcome after adjustment of any confounding variables [45, 46]. A sensible approach, which must take into consideration the individual patient clinical situation and into account the already mentioned haemostasiological parameters of erythrocytes [25, 26], would be to set a transfusion threshold with haemoglobin at 8.5-9 g/dl even for younger patients [42, 46].

6.5.3   Haemostasis

6.5.3.1 Fresh Frozen Plasma (FFP)

The use of FFP in a massive haemorrhage event is explained as an attempt to restore the flawed coagulation factors. The key guidelines recommend the use of FFP in a massive haemorrhage event and when noticeable haemostatic alterations are present (PT ratio > 1.5) [31-33]. Such recommendations however have a low rating because they are not based on solid evidence. A scrutiny of the studies available shows that the trials that analyzed the effectiveness of plasma with adequate scientific methods are few and far between. If this were a new medication, under the current stringent legislation, it would certainly not have been granted registration. The data is scarce with regard both to clinical effectiveness and to plasma infusion effects on haemostatic factors. The few studies available show that for 1 ml/kg of plasma infusion, an increase of factors levels ranging from 0.5% [47] to 2% [48] is recorded. Let us try and translate this information into a clinical situation: a patient suffered a massive haemorrhage and has received two volumes of blood consisting of erythrocyte concentrate, crystalloids and colloid, not a rare case in poly-trauma events, he/she has a factors residue level of about 15%, according to the available literature. As we have already noted, this value, in this particular *system*, is already critical because this pathology affects several aspects of haemostasis. Now let us infuse this hypothetical patient with the "traditional" 15 ml/kg of FFP:

- with a 2% recovery the factors increase by 30% and reach 45%;
- with a 0.5% recovery the factors increase by 7.5% and reach 22.5%.

The clinical differences between the first and the second situation are clear. In the first, the parameter values are harmonised to allow effective haemostasis even in the presence of interfering factors such as acidosis, hypothermia and anaemia; in the second, the clinical picture shows little change when compared to the initial situation.

The conceptual confusion that absence of evidence is tantamount to evidence of absence must be avoided. There is no evidence that FFP is of some use, the effect of the infusion is unpredictable and therefore it is of no use. Even ignoring the common clinical experience, some studies do exist proving the contrary. A Danish study on hospital haemovigilance has analysed patients receiving a massive transfusion, defined as the transfusion of >10 U of erythrocyte concentrate (EC) within 24 hours of admission or more than 30 U of EC within 7 days. [49]. The patients were subsequently divided into two categories: those who had received an adequate transfusion and those who had not, on the basis of very straightforward clinical criteria. Patients who had not received an adequate transfusion were those who had not received a platelet concentrate (PC) although they received a massive transfusion, or that had received FFP after being given 20 U of EC. Survival rate in the adequate transfusion group was 50% versus 7.7% in the non-adequate transfusion group, with p = 0.013. Following these findings, the hospital in question has adopted a "transfusion kit", comprised of 5 U of EC, 5 U of FFP and 2 of PC (equivalent to approx 30% haematocrit, 50% coagulation factors concentrate and approx $80 \cdot 10^9$/L platelets). The kit is issued automatically whenever a transfusion is deemed necessary following an acute haemorrhage [49]. A further study has looked at the benefits of this initiative and has shown that in the two years following the introduction of the kit the mortality rate at 90 days had dropped from 34.6% to 22.4% (p < 0,0001) for the same category of patients [50].

The optimum quantity of FFP to be transfused, in the form of EC/FFP ratio, has been the subject of a number of detailed studies. A study dated 2003, using a computerised model of haemostatic changes occurring during a massive haemorrhage, has shown that it is possible for as much as 70% of the blood volume to be lost before haemocomponents are transfused. In these cases, the first sign of diluted coagulopathy onset is a prolonged PT, which occurs with an 87% loss of blood volume [51]. For the patients with massive haemorrhage, the authors suggested the adoption of transfusion protocols that include 2 U of FFP for each 3 U of EC transfused, with the first 2 U of FFP being transfused simultaneously with the first EC units when the physician identifies a severe haemorrhage.

These findings have been confirmed by a subsequent study carried out on 246 patients admitted to American Military Hospitals during the Iraq conflict and diagnosed with massive haemorrhage (< 10 U of EC in 24 hours) [52]. The FFP/EC transfusion ratio was significantly linked to mortality rate: 1:1.6 in the surviving group and 1:2.3 in the non-surviving group, p < 0.001. In multivariate analysis the FFP/EC ratio was found to be associated to a survival odd ratio of 8.6, with a statistical weight analogue to the base deficit and the trauma site and severity. The study subdivided the patients into three groups according to the FFP/EC ratio: low (1:8), medium (1:1.25) and high (1:1.4). Mortality rates in the three groups were significant: 65%, 34% and 19% respectively, p < 0.05. It could be argued that bleeding in the least transfused group was so massive that time was not sufficient to provide adequate transfusion, FFP in particular. This assumption is supported by the fact that on average the patients in this group died within 2 hours. In actual fact transfused EC volume was the same in all three groups but the hourly EC transfusion volumes, as well as crystalloids volume, were significantly different.

The same findings were obtained from a later study on civilian trauma patients [53] stressing the importance of an early PC transfusion, whilst other authors specified 1:2 as the optimum FFP/EC ratio [54].

This difference of opinions, in some ways rather mystifying, is however expected in consideration of the requisites for FFP use in the absence of randomized studies and considering the high inconsistency of individual response to its transfusion. It has been proven that in patients with massive haemorrhage where FFP infusion did not manage to control bleeding, a lower increase in thrombin production was observed compared to those patients where the infusion kept the bleeding under control. In these patients, the thrombin generation lower delta was interrelated to a lower increase of fibrinogen level, which would indicate that worse outcome could somehow be linked to a lesser recovery of this haemostatic factor [55].

As we know, not only the quantity but also the timing of FFP infusion is of vital importance [51]. This concept has been explored in a subsequent study of 97 patients admitted to hospital for major trauma, no acidosis (BE > 6 mEq/L) and a transfusional requirement of > 6 U of EC within 12 hours of admission [56]. All patients were treated in ER (Emergency Room) according to the standard infusion protocol of EC and FFP with a 3:2 ratio but where the 4 FFP U were infused only after the 6 EC U. The patients were stabilised in ER in compliance with the U.S. polytrauma management protocols and transferred to the Intensive Care Unit seven hours later on average where they received a transfusion of 1:1 FFP:EC. Average INR upon admission to Intensive Care was 1.6, with a statistically significant difference between surviving and non-surviving patients of 1.5 versus 1.7 respectively, $p < 0.05$. INR upon admission to intensive care was therefore linked to mortality risk with significant statistical evidence (odds ratio 9.25 $p = 0.02$).

6.5.3.2 Other Pharmacological Approach

Desmopressin
A "must have" pharmacological product for the treatment of massive haemorrhage is Desmopressin (DDAVP), a synthetic vasopressin analogue which acts by promoting endothelial release of the Willebrand factor and by increasing glycoprotein receptors density on the platelet surface as well as the circulating level of factor VIII [57]. The efficacy of this product for the treatment of haemorrhage in patients with genetic haemostasis disorders is widely proven and documented [57, 58] but not so much in a surgical environment, where the data are somewhat contradictory [59, 60] and even less in the trauma unit environment where they are noted for their absence. At the very best, the use of DDAVP for the treatment of massive haemorrhage is therefore to be classed as complementary to the strategies so far discussed.

Antifibrinolytics
As we have already outlined, some data [28] suggest the presence of hyperfibrinolysis in trauma patients and this could justify the use of antifibronolytic preparations in such cases. Available data are unfortunately insufficient to either confirm or counter such hypothesis [61, 62]. Caution in their use is therefore recommended also in view of the potential additional risk, albeit unproven, of thromboembolism in a category of patients already at high risk.

Recombinant Activated Factor (rFVIIa)

rFVIIa , since its registration by the FDA in March 1999 for the treatment of haemophiliac patients with also factors VIII and IX inhibitors, has been hailed by many doctors as the potentially ideal pan-haemostatic agent, capable of controlling any type of bleeding even in patients free from genetic haemostatic disorders [63]. Over a few years a very impressive number of events have been put on record reporting the effective off-label use of rFVIIa for the treatment of haemorrhage in various settings, including post-surgical and poly-trauma massive bleeding [64, 65]. Such enthusiastic and general acceptance is countered by the disappointing results of randomized trials, in particular those regarding the treatment of post-trauma haemorrhage, where the only benefit appeared to be a reduction of transfusion volumes required [66]. A recent Cochrane review has quashed once and for all the expectation that rFVIIa could be the "magic bullet" to stop any kind of haemorrhage and concluded by saying that "rFVIIa has a specific role in the treatment of haemophiliac patients, but its efficacy as an haemostatic agent has yet to be confirmed. Whilst we await the results of further randomized controlled trials (RCT), the off-label use of rFVIIa should be restricted" [67]. This explanation must be acknowledged, but with some additional comments.

The randomized controlled trial is a valuable tool but of difficult application in some settings, such as the intensive care unit where, because of the patients' diversity, standardisation of population as required by applied methods is difficult to achieve. For this reason, any evaluation error in determining inclusion and exclusion criteria may lead to formally accurate conclusions that are however removed from the actual clinical situation and cannot be made to fit into a preset pattern, which is exactly the aim of a RCT.

Additionally all the physicians dealing with critical haemorrhage have learned a great deal from rFVIIa, in that they have been forced to think again about all the elements leading up to the use of this treatment, such as acidosis and hypothermia adjustment thus achieving a better management of the patient.

Fibrinogen

In the last few years the interest in this important coagulation factor has gathered momentum. The pathophysiological motivation to its use in this clinical setting is as clear as it is strong since fibrinogen plays a key role in the formation of a solid clot. Experimental models of haemorrhage in animals with induced thrombocytopenia have shown that, contrary to the expectations, the best results in terms of blood loss and survival rates were achieved administering fibrinogen rather than platelets [68]. The experimental data has significant clinical confirmation; it has in fact been proven that in women with postpartum haemorrhage, fibrinogenaemia levels < 2 g/L can predict with 100% accuracy a serious progression of the pathology [69]. This cut-off value disagrees with the 1 g/L value indicated by the current guidelines as the minimum value below which replacement therapy would be recommended [31-34]. It should however be noted that studies on clot viscoelasticity have shown the clot mechanical properties to be in line with fibrinogen concentration, without a maximum value being determined. In other words, a clot formed with a 1 g/L fibrinogen concentration is less dense than one with a concentration of 2 g/L and this in turn would be less dense than one with a concentration of 3 g/L and so forth [70]. The 1 g/L threshold value is simply related to the value below which both PT and APTT levels become altered. This would indicate that the choice of this critical value is linked to the results of laboratory tests rather than to actual haemostasis pathophysiology.

A further indication in this direction is derived from a recently published retrospective study which showed that the addition of fibrinogen (on average 2 g per patient) to the standard FFP replacement therapy in patients with massive haemorrhage and fibrinogenaemia levels below 2 g/L resulted in a substantial reduction of transfusional requirement [71].

Clearly, before being able or forced to turn these findings into general clinical procedures, a great deal of caution and prudence should be applied, ideally with the support of specifically designed clinical trials. Equally important is to continue to actively study this problem and to review the clinical procedures in the light of the indications derived from ground research and from improved understanding of underlying pathophysiology.

6.6   Protocols for the Treatment of the Haemorrhagic Patient

It is well known, as previously stated, that to date there is no single protocol for the management of patients suffering a massive haemorrhage for the simple reason that this pathology also lacks univocal definition.

Each hospital should conceive a protocol of its own, to be shared by all the relevant Specialists (Reanimation Specialists, Emergency Physicians, Transfusion Specialists, Haemostasis Specialists, Doctors of the Hospital Directorate), clearly stating the definition and the treatment of a critical haemorrhage.

Figures 6.6-6.8 illustrate a number of operational proposals derived from the experience of several Italian Centres that have dealt with this issue. The proposals also include a protocol for the use of rFVIIa since, in some instances and always applying the caution and limitations outlined in the text, the physician may regard its use as appropriate and therefore a brief outline of the recommended conduct may be valuable.

The protocols are not intended as guidelines nor as set rules on an issue of such complexity; their purpose is to motivate each hospital to develop its own haemorrhage treatment protocols in the context of the individual operational setting.

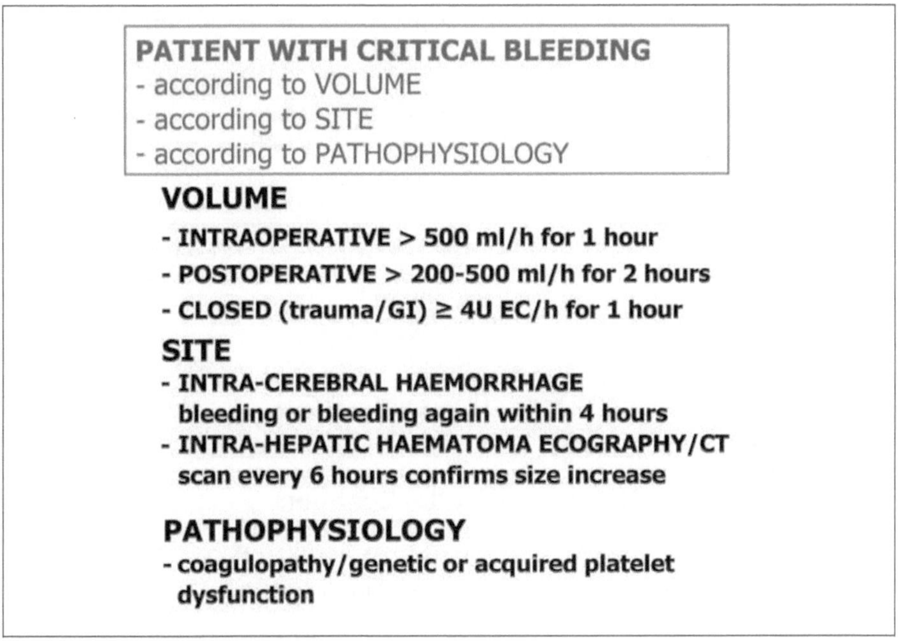

PATIENT WITH CRITICAL BLEEDING
- according to VOLUME
- according to SITE
- according to PATHOPHYSIOLOGY

VOLUME
- **INTRAOPERATIVE > 500 ml/h for 1 hour**
- **POSTOPERATIVE > 200-500 ml/h for 2 hours**
- **CLOSED (trauma/GI) ≥ 4U EC/h for 1 hour**

SITE
- **INTRA-CEREBRAL HAEMORRHAGE**
  bleeding or bleeding again within 4 hours
- **INTRA-HEPATIC HAEMATOMA ECOGRAPHY/CT**
  scan every 6 hours confirms size increase

PATHOPHYSIOLOGY
- **coagulopathy/genetic or acquired platelet**
  dysfunction

Fig. 6.6 Definition of critical bleeding

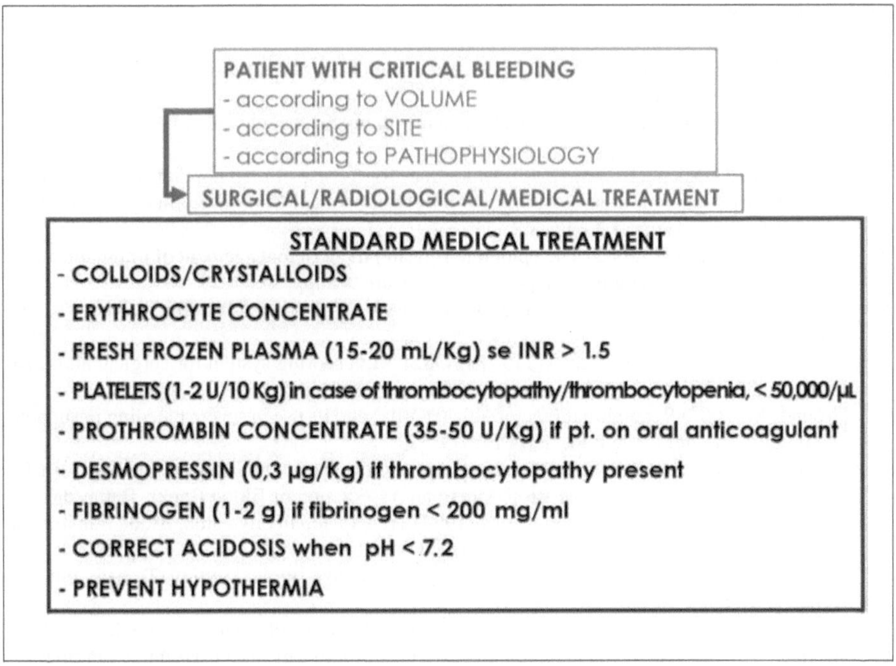

PATIENT WITH CRITICAL BLEEDING
- according to VOLUME
- according to SITE
- according to PATHOPHYSIOLOGY

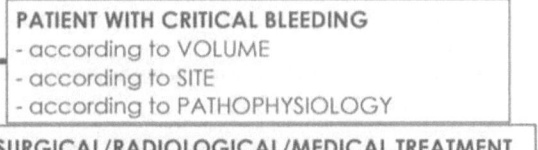

SURGICAL/RADIOLOGICAL/MEDICAL TREATMENT

STANDARD MEDICAL TREATMENT
- COLLOIDS/CRYSTALLOIDS
- ERYTHROCYTE CONCENTRATE
- FRESH FROZEN PLASMA (15-20 mL/Kg) se INR > 1.5
- PLATELETS (1-2 U/10 Kg) in case of thrombocytopathy/thrombocytopenia, < 50,000/µL
- PROTHROMBIN CONCENTRATE (35-50 U/Kg) if pt. on oral anticoagulant
- DESMOPRESSIN (0,3 µg/Kg) if thrombocytopathy present
- FIBRINOGEN (1-2 g) if fibrinogen < 200 mg/ml
- CORRECT ACIDOSIS when pH < 7.2
- PREVENT HYPOTHERMIA

Fig. 6.7 Treatment protocol for patients with critical bleeding

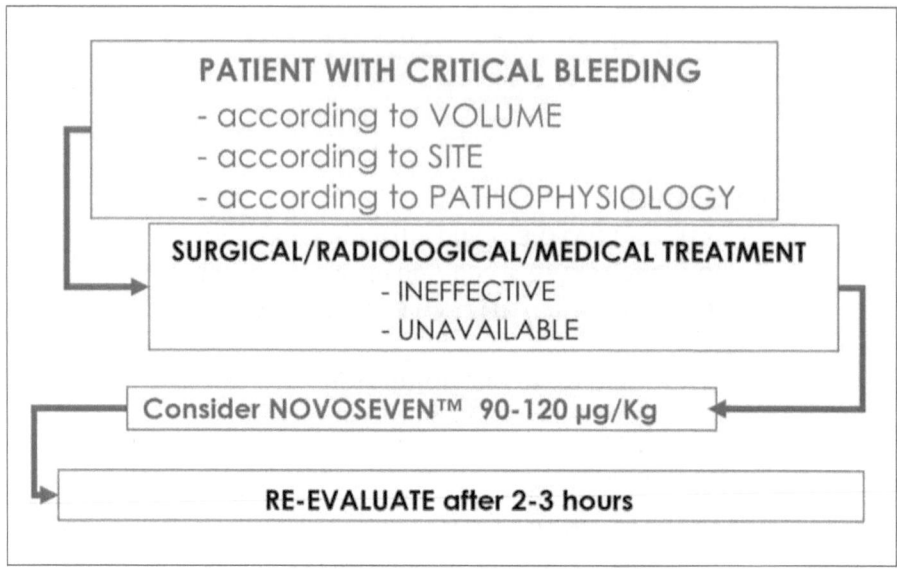

Fig. 6.8 Administration of rVIIa to patients with critical bleeding protocol

Bibliography

1. Sauaia A, Moore FA, Moore EE et al (1995) Epidemiology of trauma deaths: a reassessment.
    J Trauma 38:185-193
2. Brohi K, Singh J, Heron M, Coats T (2003) Acute traumatic coagulopathy. J Trauma 54:1127-
    1130
3. Martinowitz U, Michaelson M (2005) Guidelines for the use of recombinant activated factor
    VII (rFVIIa) in uncontrolled bleeding: a report by the Israeli Multidisciplinary rFVIIa Task
    Force. J Thromb Haemost 3:640-648
4. Kauvar DS, Wade CE (2005) The epidemiology and modern management of traumatic hem-
    orrhage: US and international perspectives. Crit Care 9(Suppl 5):S1-S9
5. Rossaint R, Cerny V, Coats TJ et al (2006) Key issues in advanced bleeding care in trauma.
    Shock 26:322-331
6. Copeland GP, Jones D, Walters M (1991) POSSUM: a scoring system for surgical audit. Br
    J Surg 78:355-360
7. Grounds M (2003) Recombinant factor VIIa (rFVIIa) and its use in severe bleeding in surgery
    and trauma: a review. Blood Reviews 17:S11-S21
8. Fakhry SM, Sheldon GF (1994) Massive transfusion in the surgical patient. In: Jeffries LC,
    Brecher ME (ed) Massive transfusion American Association of Blood Banks, Bethesda
9. Mollison PL, Engelfreit CP, Contreras M (1997) Transfusion in oligaemia. Blood transfusion
    in vlinical medicine, p 47. Blackwell Science, Oxford
10. Erber WN (2002) Massive blood transfusion in the elective surgical setting. Transfusion and
    Apheresis Science 27:83-92
11. de Gaetano G (1992) Nessuna cellula è un'isola : riflessioni sulla patogenesi della trombosi
    arteriosa. XII Congresso Nazionale Società Italiana Studio Emostasi e Trombosi. Parma, 27
    settembre-1 ottobre 1992. Abstract book, p 39

12. Colman RW, Marder VJ, Salzman EW, Hirsh J (1994) Overview of the hemostasis. In: Colman RW, Marder VJ, Salzman EW, Hirsh J (eds) Hemostasis and thrombosis. Basic Principles and clinical practice. Lippincott, Philadelphia

13. Armand R, Hess JR (2003) Treating coagulopathy in trauma patients. Transfusion Medicine Reviews 17:223-231

14. Lier H, Krep H, Schroeder S, Stuber F (2008) Preconditions of hemostasis in trauma: a review. The influence of acidosis, hypocalcemia, anemia, and hypothermia on functional hemostasis in trauma. J Trauma 65:951-960

15. Fenger-Eriksen C, Jensen M, Kristensen BS et al (2009) Fibrinogen substitution improves whole blood clot firmness following dilution with hydroxyethyl starch in bleeding patients undergoing radical cystectomy - A randomised placebo-controlled clinical trial. J Thromb Haemost Mar 5 [Epub ahead of print]

16. Wilder DM, Reid TJ, Bakaltcheva IB (2002) Hypertonic resuscitation and blood coagulation: in vitro comparison of several hypertonic solutions for their action on platelets and plasma coagulation. Thromb Res 107:255-61

17. Brummel-Ziedins K, Whelihan MF, Ziedins EG, Mann KG (2006) The resuscitative fluid you choose may potentiate bleeding. J Trauma 61:1350-1358

18. Meng ZH, Wolberg AS, Monroe DMI, Hoffman M (2003) The effect of temperature and pH on the activity of factor VIIa: implications for the efficacy of high-dose factor VIIa in hypothermic and acidotic patients. J Trauma 55:886-891

19. Raat NJ, Berends F, Verhoeven AJ et al (2005) The age of stored red blood cell concentrates at the time of transfusion. Transfus Med 15:419-423

20. Martini WZ, Dubick MA, Pusateri AE et al (2006) Does bicarbonate correct coagulation function impaired by acidosis in swine? J Trauma 61:99-106

21. Martini WZ, Dubick MA, Wade CE, Holcomb JB (2007) Evaluation of tris-hydroxymethylaminomethane on reversing coagulation abnormalities caused by acidosis in pigs. Crit Care Med 35:1568-1574

22. Johnston TD, Chen Y, Reed RL (1994) Functional equivalence of hypothermia to specific clotting factor deficiencies. J Trauma 37:413- 417

23. Martini WZ, Pusateri AE, Uscilowicz JM et al (2005) Independent contributions of hypothermia and acidosis to coagulopathy in swine. J Trauma 58:1002-1010

24. Martini WZ, Cortez DS, Dubick MA et al (2008) Thrombelastography is better than PT, APTT, and activated clotting time in detecting clinically relevant clotting abnormalities after hypothermia, hemorrhagic shock and resuscitation in pigs. J Trauma 65:535-543

25. Turitto VT, Weiss HJ (1980) Red blood cells: their dual role in thrombus formation. Science 207:541-543

26. Valeri CR, Cassidy G, Pivacek LE et al (2001) Anemia-induced increase in the bleeding time: implications for treatment of nonsurgical blood loss. Transfusion 41:977-983

27. Hardy JF, de Moerloose P, Samama M (2004) Massive transfusion and coagulopathy: pathophysiology and implications for clinical management. Can J Anesth 51:293-310

28. Levrat A, Gros A,. Rugeri L et al (2008) Evaluation of rotation thrombelastography for the diagnosis of hyperfibrinolysis in trauma patients. Br J Anaesth 100:792-797

29. Hastbacka J, Pettila V (2003) Prevalence and predictive value of ionized hypocalcemia among critically ill patients. Acta Anaesthesiol Scand 47:1264-1269

30. James MF, Roche AM (2004) Dose-response relationship between plasma ionized calcium concentration and thrombelastography. J Cardiothorac Vasc Anesth 18:581-586

31. British Committee for Standards in Haematology, Blood Transfusion Task Force (2004) Guidelines for the use of fresh-frozen plasma, cryoprecipitate and cryosupernatant. Br J Haematol 126:11-28

32. American Society of Anesthesiologists, Task Force on Perioperative Blood Transfusion and Adjuvant Therapies (2006) Practice guidelines for perioperative blood transfusion and adjuvant therapies. Anesthesiology 105:198-208

33. British Committee for Standards in Haematology Writing Group: Stainsby D, MacLennan S, Thomas D et al (2006) Guidelines on the management of massive blood loss. Br J Haematol 135:634-641

34. Erber WN, Perry DJ (2006) Plasma and plasma products in the treatment of massive haemorrhage. Best Practice & Research Clinical Haematology 19:97-112
35. Toulon P, Ozier Y, Ankri A et al (2009) Point-of-care versus central laboratory coagulation testing during haemorrhagic surgery. A multicenter study. Thromb Haemost 101:394-401
36. Luddington RJ (2005) Thrombelastography/thromboelastometry. Clin Lab Haem 27:81-90
37. Ganter MT, Hofer CK (2008) Coagulation monitoring: current techniques and clinical use of viscoelastic point-of-care coagulation devices. Anesth Analg 106:1366-1375
38. Rugeri L, Levrat A, David JS et al (2007) Diagnosis of early coagulation abnormalities in trauma patients by rotation thrombelastography. J Thromb Haemost 5:289-295
39. Spiel AO, Mayr FB, Firbas C et al (2006) Validation of rotation thrombelastography in a model of systemic activation of fibrinolysis and coagulation in humans. J Thromb Haemost 4:411-416
40. Plotkin AJ, Wade CE, Jenkins DH et al (2008) A reduction in clot formation rate and strength assessed by thrombelastography is indicative of transfusion requirements in patients with penetrating injuries. J Trauma 64:S64 -S68
41. Royston D, von Kier S (2001) Reduced haemostatic factor transfusion using heparinase-modified thrombelastography during cardiopulmonary bypass. Br J Anaesth 86:575-578
42. Busani S, Cavazzuti I, Marietta M et al (2008) Strategies to control massive abdominal bleeding. Transplantation Proceedings 40:1212-1215
43. Stahel P, Heyde C, Ertel W (2005) Current concepts of polytrauma management. Eur J Trauma 31:200-211
44. Alam HB, Burris D, DaCorta JA et al (2005) Hemorrhage control in the battlefield: role of new hemostatic agents. Mil Med 170:63-69
45. Malone DL, Dunne J, Tracy JK et al (2003) Blood transfusion, independent of shock severity, is associated with worse outcome in trauma. J Trauma 54:898-907
46. Heier HE, Bugge W, Hjelmeland K et al (2006) Transfusion vs. alternative treatment modalities in acute bleeding: a systematic review. Acta Anaesthesiol Scand 50:920
47. Blauhut B (1999) Indications for prothrombin complex concentrates in massive transfusions. Thrombosis Research 95:S63-S69
48. Spannagl M, Schramm W (1999) Replacement of coagulation factors in liver or multiple organ dysfunction. Thrombosis Research 95:S51-S56
49. Johansson PI, Hansen MB, Sorensen H (2005) Transfusion practice in massively bleeding patients: time for a change? Vox Sang 89:92-96
50. Johansson PI, Stensballe J (2009) Effect of haemostatic control resuscitation on mortality in massively bleeding patients: a before and after study. Vox Sang 96:111-118
51. Hirshberg A, Dugas M, Banez EI et al (2003) Minimizing dilutional coagulopathy in exsanguinating hemorrhage: a computer simulation. J Trauma 54:454-463
52. Borgman MA, Spinella PC, Perkins JG et al (2007) The ratio of blood products transfused affects mortality in patients receiving massive transfusions at a combat support hospital. J Trauma 63:805-813
53. Holcomb JB, Wade CE, Michalek JE et al (2008) Increased plasma and platelet to red blood cell ratios improves outcome in 466 massively transfused civilian trauma patients. Ann Surg 248:447-458
54. Kashuk JL, Moore EE,. Johnson JL et al (2008) Postinjury life threatening coagulopathy: is 1:1 Fresh Frozen Plasma: Packed Red Blood Cells the answer? J Trauma 65:261-271
55. Schols SEM, van der Meijden PEJ, van Oerle R et al (2008). Increased thrombin generation and fibrinogen level after therapeutic plasma transfusion: Relation to bleeding. Thromb Haemost 99:64-70
56. Gonzalez EA, Moore FA, Holcomb JH et al (2007) Fresh Frozen Plasma should be given earlier to patients requiring massive transfusion. J Trauma 62:112-119
57. Mannucci PM. (1998) Hemostatic drugs. New England J Med 339:245-253
58. Coppola A, Di Minno G (2008) Desmopressin in inherited disorders of platelet function. Haemophilia 14(Suppl 1):31-39

59. Carless PA, Henry DA, Moxey AJ et al (2004) Desmopressin for minimising perioperative allogeneic blood transfusion. The Cochrane Database of Systematic Reviews, Issue 1. Art. No.:CD001884.pub2.

60. Crescenzi G, Landoni G, Biondi-Zoccai G et al (2008) Desmopressin reduces transfusion needs after surgery: a meta-analysis of randomized clinical trials. Anesthesiology 109:1063-1076

61. Coats T, Roberts I, Shakur H (2004) Antifibrinolytic drugs for acute traumatic injury. Cochrane Database of Systematic Reviews, CD004896.

62. Sedrakyan A, Atkins D, Treasure T (2006) The risk of aprotinin: a conflict of evidence. Lancet 365:1376-1377

63. Hedner U (2000) NovoSeven® as a universal haemostatic agent. Blood Coagul Fibrinolysis 11:107-111

64. Martinowitz U, Kenet G, Segal E et al (2001) Recombinant activated factor VII for adjunctive hemorrhage control in trauma. J Trauma 51:431-439

65. O'Neill PA, Bluth M, Gloster ES et al (2002) Successful use of recombinant activated factor VII for trauma-associated haemorrhage in a patient without pre-existing coagulopathy. J Trauma 52:400-405

66. Boffard KD Riou B, Warren B et al for the NovoSeven Trauma Study Group (2005) Recombinant factor VIIa as adjunctive therapy for bleeding control in severely injured trauma patients: two parallel randomized, placebo-controlled, double-blind clinical trials. J Trauma 59:8-18

67. Stanworth SJ, Birchall J, Doree CJ, Hyde C (2007) Recombinant factor VIIa for the prevention and treatment of bleeding in patients without haemophilia. Cochrane Database of Systematic Reviews, Issue 2. Art.No.:CD005011

68. Velik-Salchner C, Haas T, Innerhofer P et al (2007) The effect of fibrinogen concentrate on thrombocytopenia. J Thromb Haemost 5:1019-1025

69. Charbit B, Mandelbrot L, Samain E et al for the PPH Study Group (2007) The decrease of fibrinogen is an early predictor of the severity of postpartum hemorrhage. J Thromb Haemost 5: 266-273

70. Dempfle CE, Kälsch T, Elmas E et al (2008) Impact of fibrinogen concentration in severely ill patients on mechanical properties of whole blood clots. Blood Coagulation and Fibrinolysis 19:765-770

71. Fenger-Eriksen C, Lindberg-Larsen M, Christensen AQ et al (2008) Fibrinogen concentrate substitution therapy in patients with massive haemorrhage and low plasma fibrinogen concentrations. Br J Anaesth 101:769-773.

Hypercapnic Acidosis in Protective Mechanical Ventilation (a Tolerated Compromise or Another Means of Protection?)

7

Biagio Allaria

7.1 Introduction

As Laffey accurately pointed out ten years ago [1], we are all used to thinking that the range of normal values commonly accepted for healthy individuals are also useful for critical patients, but this approach is certainly not based on reality. For example, administering oxygen to premature neonates to achieve "normal" PaO_2 levels may lead to retinopathy and bronchopulmonary dysplasia; giving transfusions to critical patients trying to reach normal haematocrit levels may increase mortality rates; and aiming for normal pressure levels in patients with multiple trauma may reduce their chances of survival. We should therefore not forget that elevated $PaCO_2$ levels in critical patients (or even maintaining lower levels than normal), can have harmful effects.

The truth is that since we have known for more than 15 years that low-Vt ventilation and low pressure in the airways reduces damage to the lungs caused by mechanical ventilation, it is agreed that this mechanical action has the advantage of reducing mortality rates in the treatment of acute respiratory distress syndrome (ARDS). All too often, however, this type of ventilation causes hypercapnia and therefore acidosis, or at least makes it possible, and as such is considered a minor evil when compared with the advantages obtained with so-called protective mechanical ventilation. Anyone who has examined the international literature in detail (in reality, most studies have been conducted in animals species using isolated and perfused lungs), would not think that hypercapnic acidosis could have a protective role in patients

B. Allaria (✉)
Past Director of Critical Care Department
Istituto Nazionale per lo Studio e la Cura dei Tumori - National Cancer Institute, Milan, Italy
e-mail: biagio.allaria@tiscali.it

with respiratory insufficiency and would certainly not consider it to be a minor evil to be tolerated.

In this chapter we shall see how, in reality, respiratory acidosis can have a protective effect not only on the lungs but also on other organs and, by understanding that patients with ARDS often die not from hypoxaemia but from multiple organ failure (MOF), it is worth considering as a treatment strategy that can protect a number of organs.

However, without wanting to refute the importance of mechanical ventilation as a protective measure, it cannot be denied that recent improvements in the survival of ARDS patients are not only attributed to this but also to other therapeutic approaches that have been perfected over time. This includes today's focus on fluid replacement, more incisive nursing (including pronation), more comprehensive support for patients with renal insufficiency, appropriate nutritional supplements and pulmonary circulation during, amongst other things, mechanical ventilation.

Therefore, at the end of this chapter readers may be convinced that in addition to the procedures listed above, hypercapnic acidosis may also play a protective role, and that recent successes may also, in part, be attributed to it. However, since hyperventilation was frequently employed in the past, and this frequently caused patients to develop hypocapnic alkalosis, we must assume that abandoning this strategy is clearly the right step to take.

In reality, it has long been known that hypocapnic alkalosis may itself be the cause of pulmonary damage [2]. More than thirty years ago the negative effect of induced hypocapnia was already demonstrated in patients with chronic obstructive pulmonary disease (COPD) [3] in whom compliance decreased, and it was shown that in animal studies [4] hypocapnia increased pulmonary microvascular permeability and reduced the production of surfactants [5].

In addition to this we know that alkalosis causes a left-shift in the oxygen-haemoglobin dissociation curve, making it harder for oxygen to be supplied to tissues, which are less perfused in the event of hypocapnia due to the resulting vasoconstriction.

Those who work in neurosurgery are particularly aware of the negative effects of hypocapnia. The harmful effects on the brain that prophylactic hyperventilation causes in patients with cranial injuries [6] are well known, and those involved in clinical trials for ischemic strokes know that this disorder is more serious in hyperventilated animals [7]. Thus, anyone who deals with closely related disorders will know that neurological damage at high altitudes a long time after exposure is not due to hypoxia but rather to hypocapnia.

These examples aim to show that abandoning hyperventilation can be an advantageous strategy not only because it enables damage from pulmonary hyperdistention to be reduced but also, at least in part, because it eliminates a dangerous effect: hypocapnic alkalosis.

7.2   Does Hypercapnic Acidosis Protect the Lungs from Damage?

Once again we shall refer to the study conducted by Laffey, the Head of the Physiology Department at University College Dublin. The objective of this study was to observe pulmonary behaviour in rats with acute lung injury (ALI) induced by endotoxins, with or without previous treatment with elevated $FiCO_2$ that led to hypercapnic acidosis.

The first question was: does hypercapnic acidosis protect the lungs from damage caused by endotoxins? The study objective was clear, namely to show that even in ARDS patients with sepsis (one of the most common disorders) hypercapnic acidosis can have a protective function. The findings were positive: in rats previously treated with hypercapnic acidosis, the fall in PaO_2 was lower, compliance improved, and neutrophil infiltration and the histological markers of pulmonary damage decreased. There was also less production of oxidants.

The next question was: how does hypercapnic acidosis protect the lungs from endotoxin damage? Lipopolysaccharide, an endotoxin in Gram-negative microorganisms, begins its harmful effect by stimulating a specific receptor of the innate immune system (toll-like receptor 4). Laffey's work has shown that hypercapnic acidosis is effective in preventing and curing damage caused by activation of this receptor. Moreover, it may be interesting to know that hypercapnic acidosis also has a protective role by blocking the production of peroxynitrite (the result of a reaction between NO and superoxide radicals), which in turn causes the nitrification of amino acids, such as the formation of nitrothyroxine from thyroxine.

These reactions significantly alter the protein structures of the lungs, to such an extent that in patients with sepsis great importance is given to the confirmation of nitrothyroxine as a marker of pulmonary damage. Therefore, hypercapnic acidosis does not protect the lungs by blocking this pathway: that is, it does not block nitrification of amino acids in pulmonary proteins due to peroxynitrite. In fact, a product of this mechanism, nitrothyroxine, is not only decreased in rats previously treated with hypercapnic acidosis but also increased.

The third question was: is it hypercapnia that protects the lungs or acidosis, or both? Previous studies have analysed these two factors separately, and in some ways it would seem that acidosis plays a major role in generating the protective effect. Laffey's earlier study [8] is important in this respect; it also involved rats but used a different method of producing pulmonary damage (ischemia-reperfusion) and showed that damage was greater if, in cases of hypercapnic acidosis, acidosis was compensated by $NaHCO_3$. Acidosis itself therefore has a protective role.

One limitation of this study, however, when extrapolating the results to clinical situations, is that perfused lungs were used that were isolated from the general circulation. The study did not take into account the possible effects of hypercapnic acidosis on the general circulation and on pulmonary circulation itself.

However, the fact that intracellular acidosis has a protective effect on pulmonary damage also appears to have been ascertained in earlier studies that had already shown that both metabolic and respiratory acidosis have a protective effect, albeit markedly higher with respiratory acidosis.

This is probably due to the very high availability of CO_2 inside cells, leading to the very effective production of H^+ ($CO_2 + H_2O = H^+ + HCO_3$). In metabolic acidosis, H^+ are extracellular since cell membranes are relatively impermeable under stress. In the event of hypercapnic acidosis, intracellular acidosis is therefore considerably greater than metabolic acidosis and this is probably the reason for the increased effectiveness of protection from hypercapnic acidosis.

There is, however, an obstacle to this argument: $NaHCO_3$ administration creates an overproduction of CO_2, which spreads into the cells and causes intracellular acidosis. To what extent does the administration of $NaHCO_3$ reduce the protective effect of hypercapnic acidosis? It would seem that this damage is linked to the obstruction of Na transport channels and therefore the passage of water from the alveolar epithelium to the interstitium, with a resulting build-up of liquid in the alveoli.

The harmful effect of $NaHCO_3$ would therefore be linked not to a reduction in protective intracellular acidosis, which in fact increases, but to a diverse mechanism that leads to deterioration of pulmonary oedema.

Some words should be said about the effect of hypercapnic acidosis on pulmonary circulation. Here too, it is necessary to distinguish between the effect of hypercapnia and acidosis. Hypercapnia is a potent pulmonary vasodilator [9] but acidosis, on the other hand, is a vasoconstrictor.

Using the data from Laffey's study, it can be seen that stopping acidosis with $NaHCO_3$ triggers a pulmonary vasodilator effect with hypercapnia alone.

In the past there was often talk of hypercapnic vasoconstriction which, like hypoxic vasoconstriction, would be useful in diverting the flow from the least ventilated alveoli to the most ventilated ones, thereby helping to reduce the shunt fraction.

If Laffey's data and similar results obtained by Viles more than forty years ago [10] are correct, so-called "hypercapnic vasoconstriction" should fact be called "acidotic vasoconstriction".

It is, however, important, from a practical perspective, to consider hypercapnic acidosis wholly as a pulmonary vasoconstrictor that exerts its action on precapillary arterioles by increasing mean pulmonary arterial pressure (PAP) but with no increase in wedge pressure (WP). Since the formula commonly used to calculate pulmonary vascular resistance (PVR) with Swan-Ganz catheters is:

$$PVR = \frac{80 \cdot (PAP\ mean\ -\ WP)}{CO}$$

it is clear that an increase in mean PAP with low WP (as is commonly the case in patients with ARDS) leads to a rise in PVR with an increase in precapillary arteriolar resistance.

Perhaps the most comprehensive study of the effects of hypercapnia on pulmonary circulation and the heart was conducted by Kiely et al [11] in healthy young volunteers, using a Doppler ultrasound control method. The volunteers were tested before and after inhaling a CO_2-rich mixture with the aim of achieving hypercapnia of 55-60 mmHg with the measurement of numerous useful parameters to assess the response of pulmonary circulation, peripheral circulation and the heart. In the systemic circulation an increase in CO, SV, HR, SBP, DBP and MAP (medium arterial pressure) has been observed with a slight and insignificant reduction in SVR. Changes of this kind were already observed fifty years ago by Price [11] and thirty-five years ago by Cullen [12]. However, whereas previous experiments on isolated hearts demonstrated a depressant effect for hypercapnia [13], in this study no such effect was found. In fact, increased aortic flow and peak flow did not change with hypercapnia, meaning that this neither reduced nor increased myocardial contractility.

The meaning of this is unclear: the effect of hypercapnia on the central and autonomic nervous systems (with increased vasomotor tone and amine release) cancels out the direct depressant effect of hypercapnia. This indirect effect has been known for many years [14, 15].

An interesting observation in this study was QT dispersion on the ECG (variations between minimum and maximum values). This parameter was changed by hypercapnia and, together with the increase in the circulation of accompanying amines, promoted rhythm disorders. Such observations turn one's thoughts immediately to respiratory situations that are accompanied by fatal arrhythmias in which hypercapnia could play a prominent role, such as sleep apnoea and COPD.

An interesting study that analysed circulation patterns in humans with hypercapnia was published in 1991 by Ebata et al. [16] from the University of Tokyo. The authors monitored haemodynamic behaviour in patients who were possible organ donors and in whom diagnosis of brain death led to the prediction of apnoea with hypercapnia; their objective was to evaluate the presence and absence of bulbar respiratory responses to hypercapnia. Patients were detached from ventilator and apnoeic oxygenation was maintained with pure O_2 administered via a catheter inserted into the orotracheal tube; they maintained in apnoea until reaching $PaCO_2 > 60$ mmHg. In these conditions the usual haemodynamic parameters were recorded: CO, PVR and mean PAP increased significantly whereas mean AP, WP and RAP (right atrial pressure) remained unchanged. The plasma noradrenaline concentrations of three patients were measured, which consistently indicated an increase in the hypercapnic phase. The course of the parameters was typical for an increase in pulmonary arteriolar resistance without involvement of the right ventricle (right atrial pressure was unchanged). Cardiac depression could not be demonstrated and there was in fact an increase (more CO). The direct vasodilator effect of CO_2 could therefore not be proven, probably due to the possibility of a medullar adrenergic response (the central vasomotor pathway in these patients having been blocked by existing serious brain injury). For the same reason, myocardial depression directly resulting from CO_2 could not be proven either.

To a significant extent, therefore, hypercapnic acidosis in humans generally does not lead to myocardial depression due to medullar and central nervous responses (if the vasomotor centre is intact), thus tending to increase cardiac supply. In the lungs there is an increase in pulmonary arteriolar resistance that is well tolerated in the right ventricle and may be useful in pushing the flow towards better ventilated parts of the lungs and thus helping to reduce the shunt fraction.

To underline the fact that this is usual in the circulation in response to hypercapnia, there are situations in which behaviour can be very diverse.

For example, it has been shown that when medullar responses are restricted by spinal blockade [17], hypercapnia causes a significant fall in CO and arterial pressure, thereby resulting in a whole range of direct vasodilator and myocardial depressant effects.

With this in mind it is easy to think what can happen to a patient with COPD undergoing surgery with spinal anaesthesia if $PaCO_2$ increases for any reason, such as excessive and inappropriate sedation.

7.3   The Role of Hypercapnic Acidosis in Pulmonary Oedema and Mechanisms for Preventing and Repairing Damage

Alveoli have a total surface area of 143 m², 95% of which is covered with type 1 alveolar cells (AT1 cells) and 5% with type 2 cells (AT2 cells). The close connection between alveoli and capillaries promotes the exchange of gases but is a barrier for fluids and proteins in the interstitium and vessels, meaning that the alveoli remain relatively dry.

Between cells, whether alveolar cells or endothelial cells, there are junctions that form "pores" with a radius of 0.5-0.9 μm for the alveolar epithelium and 6.5-7.5 μm for the vascular epithelium. Therefore the greater resistance to the flow of water and proteins is not in the vessels but the alveoli where the pores are smaller, and this is an area where the alveoli are usually dry.

However, if fluid enters the alveoli, an active pump system enables it to be transported to the interstitium. In both AT1 and AT2 cells there is an active sodium transport system from the apex to the base and the interstitium (Na/K-ATPase). Until a few years ago this process was attributed only to AT2 cells but only because they were easier to isolate and study.

Now, thanks to the work of Ridge [18], it is known that this is also possible for AT1 cells, which, as we have seen, are the components that are much more widely represented in alveoli (95% versus 5%). In Ridge's study he concludes that the α_2-isoform of Na/K-ATPase in AT1 cells is responsible for 60% of fluid absorption by β-adrenergic stimulation (it has been known for some time that β_2-stimulants contribute to alveolar fluid clearance). It has been shown that β_2-stimulants such as terbutaline, salmeterol and salbutamol stimulate the uptake of sodium from the apex of alveolar cells and transport it towards the base from which α_2 Na/K-0ATPase transfers it together with H_2O to the interstitium.

This seems to be the cause of the increase in pulmonary lymphatic drainage that follows the use of β_2-stimulants. It appears, however, that long-term exposure to β_2-stimulants eventually worsens fluid clearance from the lungs and this worsening may be linked to a progressive reduction in the number of β_2-receptor cells. This does not take away from the fact that β_2-stimulants can be recommended for promoting pulmonary fluid clearance.

Hypoxia disturbs both intracellular transport of sodium and the passage via Na/K-ATPase from the basal membrane to the interstitium, and therefore leads to a worsening of alveolar fluid clearance.

In cases of oedema caused by increased hydrostatic pressure (acute or chronic cardiac insufficiency) with an intact alveolar-capillary barrier, patients receiving appropriate assistance and mechanical ventilation have a surprisingly quick alveolar fluid clearance rate. Current practice is to implement rapid resolution of acute pulmonary oedema with mechanical ventilation in such cases. Experimental studies on this type of pulmonary oedema have shown that intracellular sodium transport mechanisms via epithelial sodium channels (EnaC) and the transfer of basal membranes to the interstitium are both intact.

In ALI these mechanisms are damaged and therefore fluid clearance is obstructed. There is a correlation between the level of damage to these transport mechanisms and mortality [19].

Damage to sodium and water transport mechanisms is, however, possible, especially in episodes of recurrent acute pulmonary oedema (APO), even in the case of cardiac insufficiency, when the barrier is generally intact. Inflammatory mediators can, in fact, be released in such cases, damaging the transport mechanism and promoting successive episodes of APO even without a considerable increase in hydrostatic pressure. These mediators are similarly released by distension of the left atrium and are responsible for the inexplicably frequent recurrence of APO in heart disease patients who apparently have good compensation.

The mechanism that causes pulmonary oedema in patients with multiple trauma and haemorrhage is interesting. Following haemorrhage, neutrophils build up in the lungs and release oxidant radicals and β-interleukin. Moreover, NO synthase production is increased and results in the release of NO (perhaps from pulmonary macrophages). All this alters the transport of intraepithelial and epithelial-interstitial sodium.

In patients with sepsis there is a real and genuine problem of endothelial and epithelial damage probably linked to proteases released by neutrophils, from oxygen radicals and bacterial products. For example, it has been seen that Gram-negative microorganisms that produce proteases increase the permeability of the barrier more than Gram-negative microorganisms that do not produce proteases.

Mechanical ventilation can damage these mechanisms by harming the alveolar-capillary interface [20], affecting permeability [21] and causing oedemas [22, 23].

It is now clear that protective ventilation with low Vt and low pressure in the airways may have an advantage in reducing mechanical damage, but there is still debate about whether hypercapnic acidosis, which mainly accompanies this type of ventilation, is itself protective; as we have seen, there are many studies that support his notion. Yet clarification is still required to shed light on the objectives of such situations, not only in terms of preventing damage (in which case protective ventilation and hypercapnic acidosis play a positive role), but also to facilitate reparative processes.

A recent study by Doerr et al. [24] of the Mayo Clinic contains interesting data despite being conducted in rats. The authors ventilated animals with high Vt (40 mL/kg for every 20 minutes) but with various $FiCO_2$ levels in order to have three categories of rats: normocapnic, hypocapnic and hypercapnic. In all cases the lungs were perfused with substances that became fluorescent under blue light and to which the alveolar-capillary barrier is usually impermeable. The passing of these substances from vessels to the alveolar epithelium indicated damage that could be defined as permanent or transient according to when the marker was administered. Damage was defined as permanent only when the marker was infused at the end of harmful ventilation; it was defined as transient or permanent when this occurred during ventilation. The main changes to the barrier were observed in hypocapnic animals; the least common in hypercapnic animals. This observation is in line with those of other authors to whom we have already referred, and who have demonstrated the protective effect of hypercapnic acidosis towards the alveolar-capillary barrier in animals undergoing harmful ventilation. But what is interesting and fairly new is the discovery that damage repair is 25% less effective in animals with hypercapnia compared to those with normocapnia. Therefore, according to these experiments, hypercapnia slows transient damage but obstructs the repair of damage, and therefore the percentage of necrotic cells ends up being higher in hypercapnic patients than in normocapnic ones.

This should not discourage the use of protective ventilation with hypercapnic acidosis because the decrease in transient damage by reducing the number of affected cells also reduces the number of cells that may trigger a prolonged inflammatory response likely to involve neighbouring cells and amplify damage to the barrier.

Above all, the understanding that hypercapnic acidosis slows the reparative processes should not encourage the use of bicarbonate, which produces CO_2 and later reduces pH in alveolar epithelial cells that are impermeable to the transepithelial flow of bicarbonate but permeable to CO_2. In addition, as we said before, the administration of bicarbonate blocks sodium intraepithelial transport channels and its transfer from the base of the epithelium to the interstitium using α_2 Na/K-ATPase compromises alveolar fluid clearance [25]. For many years the harmful effect that bicarbonate has on anaesthetised and ven-tilated animals by causing hypercapnic acidosis has been known for many years [26, 27].

In the extensive literature, albeit lacking a unanimous consensus, there seems to be a considerable acceptance of hypercapnic acidosis accompanying protective ventilation, but we cannot overlook its effects, which, if present, require a revision of the ventilation strategy. In particular we refer to cardiac arrhythmias and the potential deterioration of pulmonary oedema.

We have in fact already seen how hypercapnic acidosis causes changes in QT dispersion and can create a predisposition to arrhythmic events. However, deaths from probable arrhythmic causes are more often recorded in patients with hypercapnia such as COPD and sleep apnoea [28, 29].

Another situation in which the ventilation strategy may be revised is marked by deterioration of pulmonary oedema as well as an expected reduction in pro-tective ventilation. Worsening of pulmonary fluid clearance in patients with hypercapnia has in fact been described independently of acidosis [30].

Finally, there is no consensus, especially on the importance of the tolerabil-ity level for acidosis and in particular on the cautious use of bicarbonate, which is still under discussion. We have repeatedly said that the protective effect of pulmonary damage due to hypercapnic acidosis is linked to acidosis rather than to hypercapnia: stopping acidosis risks bringing the effect of acidosis to an end and, by worsening intracellular acidosis in the alveolar epithelium, there is a risk of harmful mechanisms in which epithelial and epithelio-interstitial trans-port of alveolar fluids is obstructed.

It is probably for this reason that bicarbonate is not recommended, but in patients with serious acidosis it is permitted by the ARDS Network Study [31].

It is not easy to define the critical pH limit under which cautious bicarbon-ate use is justified if it is not possible to change the ventilation strategy or extra-corporeal CO_2 clearance. In the previously mentioned study on hypercapnic acidosis induced by the apnoea test in patients with brain death, no changes in haemodynamic stability were observed up to pH 7.17 ± 0.002 (with $PaCO_2$ at 60-80 mmHg).

Furthermore, the decision to use more or less bicarbonate depends on the patient and not only on the critical pH level. For instance, in the case of a patient with endocranial hypertension or at risk of developing it, hypercapnic acidosis can trigger cerebral perfusion. In this case pH levels should not be maintained too low, and bicarbonate may be administered cautiously. On the other hand, bicarbonate causes a later increase in CO_2, and it was demonstrat-ed more than ten years ago by Cardenas [32] that if acidosis is stopped, endocranial pressure does not increase despite hypercapnia. In this work Cardenas stated that the use of bicarbonate was acceptable for pH < 7.20 and even < 7.30 in patients with endocranial hypertension, possibly using a mixture of 5% sodium bicarbonate and sodium carbonate that was shown to cause a slight rise in CO_2 compared to bicarbonate alone.

7.4   Can the Extent of Hypercapnia in Protective Ventilation Be Limited?

Partial CO_2 pressure (PCO_2) is the result of the following factors:

a. $PCO_2 = K \cdot (VCO_2/AV) + FiCO_2$

where: VCO_2 = CO_2 production; AV = alveolar ventilation; $FiCO_2$ = fractional inspired CO_2. AV corresponds to total ventilation minus the dead space, i.e.:

b. $AV = Vt - Vd/Vt = Vt \cdot (1-Vd/Vt)$

where Vt is total ventilation and Vd/Vt is the dead space. Combining equations (**a**) and (**b**) gives:

$$PCO_2 = K \cdot VCO_2/Vt \, (1-Vd/Vt) + FiCO_2$$

Therefore the determining factors of an increase in PCO_2 are

- $VCO2$ = increased production;
- $1/VT$ = reduced ventilation;
- Vd/Vt = negative pulmonary perfusion (increase in dead space);
- $PiCO2$ = increased $FiCO2$.

Since hypercapnia in protective ventilation is substantially due to a fall in Vt, in order to limit it we can act only on VCO_2 and Vd/Vt since we cannot increase Vt without detriment to the protective ventilation strategy.

It will therefore be seen that we have the possibility of reducing these two factors. CO_2 is the product of oxidant metabolism and the amount is proportional to O_2 consumption (VO_2), using this equation:

$$VCO_2 = RQ \cdot VO_2$$

where RQ is the respiratory quotient, which is 0.7 for lipids, 0.85 for proteins and 1 for carbohydrates.

This equation clearly shows that food plays a significant role in the production of CO_2 and that too many carbohydrates should be avoided. From the same equation it can be seen that the second factor that contributes to CO_2 production is VO_2. Here too, the most common causes, such as fever, psychomotor agitation and difficulty breathing should be limited.

CO_2, however, is not only produced with the oxidative cycle but also, during tissue hypoxia, by ATP and ADP hydrolysis. The resulting formation of acids leads to a release of H^+ that is stopped by HCO_3^- with the formation of CO_2 and H_2O:

$$H^+ + HCO_3^- \rightarrow H_2O + CO_2$$

The formation of CO_2 that follows hypoxia does not lead to hypercapnia if normal ventilation is preserved but in cases of protective ventilation, for example, it may be a cause of hypercapnia and acidosis that exceeds tolerated levels. The increase in tissular CO_2 in such cases is considered to be a sign of dysoxia and has opened the way to suitable monitoring systems to identify it, such as gastric and sublingual tonometry, with $\Delta a - v\ CO_2$ [33, 34, 35].

The importance of increased CO_2 during tissue dysoxia is, however, controversial since CO_2 is produced either by aerobic or anaerobic metabolism and increases in tissues as well as by stagnation if perfusion is compromised [35].

Vallet [36] showed ten years ago that by inducing hypoxic tissue dysoxia in animals, $\Delta a - v\ CO_2$ remained unchanged; however, it increased threefold in cases of ischemic dysoxia caused by compromised perfusion [36].

The increase in venous and tissular CO_2 is not therefore generally the expression of dysoxia but of perfusion damage. This observation has been confirmed by other authors such as Nevière [37] and Dubin [38] who have found the same discrepancy between hypoxic changes and hypoperfusional changes in the intestines in pigs and sheep.

There is therefore a fairly good consensus that increases in venous and tissular CO_2 during dysoxia may be linked to ischemic causes rather than a hypoxic causes.

This understanding is shared by Gutierrez [39], who has developed a mathematical model for the study of CO_2 behaviour in tissues and veins in patients with hypoxia and hyperperfusion.

Therefore, due to the importance of perfusion in triggering CO_2 production, it is vital that it is optimised when implementing a protective ventilation strategy with low Vt, in order not to combine hypoventilation-induced hypercapnia with a hypercapnic component that is theoretically avoidable and linked to tissue hypoperfusion. In this sense it is also necessary to adopt this strategy to optimise pulmonary perfusion with the intention of not promoting an increase in Vd/Vt, which, as we have seen, is one of the determining factors for hypercapnia.

In reality, in recent years we have been concerned mainly with monitoring poorly ventilated or non-ventilated or non-perfused areas, controlling the shunt fraction (QS/QT) and by paying little attention to the opposite developments in areas that are ventilated but poorly perfused (Vd/Vt). Fortunately, the most recent reports have led us to shift our attention to this, even following the observation that mortality in ARDS patients is correlated with the course of Vd/Vt [40]. It will also be necessary to take this aspect into account in PEEP optimisation strategies.

Therefore, the measures to be taken to avoid excess levels of hypercapnia and acidosis in patients with protective ventilation can be summarised as moderate use of carbohydrates, a reduction in excess VO_2 related to fever, psychomotor agitation and difficulty breathing, and finally close control of tissue perfusion in general and pulmonary perfusion in particular.

7.5   Conclusions

Since 1990, when Hickling described the use of ventilation with low Vt and limited pressure in the airways of adults with ARDS [41], the hypercapnic acidosis that accompanies this "protective" strategy has been considered a "minor evil" to be accepted along with the benefits obtained from ventilation that enables a reduction in mechanical damage to the lungs from conventional mechanical ventilation.

Later works have also had the benefit not only of confirming this but also of greatly extending the method of protective ventilation to worldwide intensive care facilities. For example, studies by Amato and Carvalho [42, 43] have always regarded hypercapnic acidosis to be a collateral effect of treatment and therefore (in the words of Amato) a "variable of secondary importance" [44].

More or less during the same period, however, the number of studies on the effects of hypercapnic acidosis on the lungs in patients with ARDS has increased, mostly with animal studies that, as we have seen, contribute to a growing literature that considers hypercapnic acidosis to be not so much an adverse effect as a protective feature that can be summed up as a new ventilation strategy.

In 1999, in the work mentioned above that was published in *The Lancet*, Laffrey was able to take into consideration the possibility of inducing hypercapnia in critical patients to initiate a new organ protection strategy. This is perhaps going too far, but it is a sign of the "reversal" of convictions that have formed in recent years.

We do not feel we have reached this point, nor have we accepted extreme levels of hypercapnic acidosis. Instead, it seems rational to accept reasonable $PaCO_2$ and pH levels with the same precautions as those described in the previous chapter paragraph 7.4 to avoid extreme levels for hypercapnic acidosis, which we are all still wary of, and rightly so.

Bibliography

1. Laffey GJ, Kavanagh BP (1999) Carbon dioxide and the critically ill-too little of a good thing? Lancet 354:1283-1286
2. Garland JS, Buck RK, Allred EN et al (1995) Hypocarbia before surfactant therapy appears to increase bronchopulmonary dysplasia risk in infants with respiratory distress syndrome. Arch Ped Adolesc Med 149:617-622
3. Cutillo A, Omboni E, Parondi R et al. (1974) Effects of hypocapnia on pulmonary mechanics in normal subjects and in patients with COPD. Am Rev Resp Dis 110:25-33
4. Raynolds AM, Zadow SP, Sciochitano R et al (1992) Hypocapnia increases microvascular leakage in the guinea pig trachea. Am Rev Resp Dis 145:80-84
5. Oyarzun MJ, Donoso P, Quijade D (1986) Role of hypocapnia in the alveolar surfactant increase induced by free fatty acid intravenous infusion in the rabbit. Respiration 49:187-194
6. Mulzelaar JP, Marmarou A, Word JD et al (1991) Adverse effects of prolonged hyperventilation in patients with severe head injury: a randomized trial. J Neurosurg. 75:731-739
7. Vannucci RF, Towfligh J, Heitjan DF et al (1995) Carbon dioxide protects the perinatal brain from hypoxic-ischemic damage: an experimental study in the immature rat. Pediatrics 95:868-874

8. Laffey JG, Honan D, Hopkins N et al (2004) Hypercapnic acidosis attenuates endotoxin-induced acute lung injury. Am J Resp Crit Care Me 169:46-56
9. Laffey JG, Engelberts D, Kavanagh B (2000) Buffering hypercapnic acidosis worsens ALI. Am J Resp Crit Care Med 161:141-146
10. Viles PH, Shepard JT (1968) Evidence for a dilator action of carbon dioxide on the pulmonary vessels of the cat. Circ Resp 22:325-332
11. Price HL (1960) Effects of carbon dioxide on the cardiovascular system. Anesthesiology 21:652-53
12. Cullen DJ, Enger EI (1974) Cardiovascular effects of carbon dioxide in man. Anesthesiology 41:345-349
13. Williams FM (1955) Individual effects of CO2, bicarbonate and pH on the electrical and mechanical activity of isolated rabbit auricles. J. Physiol 129:90-110
14. Cross BA, Silver IA (1962) Central activation of sympathadrenal system by hypoxia and hypercarbia. J. Andocrinol 24:91-93
15. Downing SE, Siegal JH (1963) Baroceptor and chemoreceptor influences on sympathetic discharge to the heart. Am J Physiol 204:471-79
16. Ebata T, Watanabe Y, Amaha K et al (1991) Hemodynamic changes during the apnoea test for diagnosis of brain death. Can J Anaesth 33:436-440
17. Kimura K (1978) Experimental studies on cerebro-spinal anesthesia. Masni 27:1059-1070
18. Ridge KM, Olivera WG, Soldias F et al (2003) Alveolar type 1 cells express the α_2 Na/K-ATPase, which contribute to lung liquid clearance. Circ Res 92:453-460
19. Matthay MA, Folkesson HG, Clerici C (2002) Lung epithelial fluid transport and resolution of pulmonary edema. Physiol Rev 82:569-600
20. Fu Z, Costello ML, Tsukimoto H et al (1992) High lung volume increases stress failure in pulmonary capillaries. J Appl Physiol 73:123-133
21. Carlton DP, Cummings JJ, Scheerer RG et al (1990). Lung overexpansion increases pulmonary microvascular protein permeability in young lambs. J Appl Physiol 69:577-583
22. Parker JC, Hernandez LA, Longenecker GL et al (1990) Lung edema caused by high peak inspiratory pressure in dogs: role of increased microvascular filtration pressure and permeability. Am Rev Resp Dis 142:321-328
23. Dreyfuss D, Saumon G (1993) Role of tidal volume, FRC and end-inspiratory volume in the development of pulmonary edema followed mechanical ventilation. Am Rev Resp Dis 148:1194-1203
24. Doerr CH, Gaijc O, Berrios JC et al (2005) Hypercapnic acidosis impairs plasma membrane wound realizing in ventilation-injured lungs. Am J Resp Crit Care Med 171:1371-1377
25. Joseph D, Dimiri O, Zhang XL et al (2002) Alveolar epithelial ion and fluid transport: polarity of alveolar epithelial cell acid-base permeability. Am J Physiol Lung Cell Med Physiol 282:L675-L683
26. Nishikawa T (1993) Acute haemodynamic effect of sodium bicarbonate in canine respiratory or metabolic acidosis. Br J Anaesth 70:196-200
27. Tanaka M, Nishikawa T (1997) Acute haemodynamic effect of sodium bicarbonate administration in respiratory and metabolic acidosis in anesthetized dogs. Anaesth Int Care 25:615-620
28. McNicholas WT, Bonsignore MR (2007) Sleep apnea as an independent risk factor for cardiovascular disease: current evidence, basic mechanism, and research priorities. Eur Resp J 29:156-178
29. Sin DD, Man SF (2005) Chronic obstructive pulmonary disease as a risk factor for cardiovascular morbidity and mortality. Proc Am Ther Soc 2:8-11
30. Chen J, Secuona E, Briva A et al (2008) Carbonic antydrase II and alveolar fluid absorption during hypercapnia. Am J Resp Cell Med Biol 38:32-37
31. The Acute Respiratory Distress Syndrome Network (2003) Ventilation with lower tidal volume as compared with traditional tidal volumes for acute lung injury and acute respiratory distress syndrome. N Eng J Med 342:1301-1308
32. Cardenas V, Zwischenberger J, Tao W (1996) Correction of blood pH attenuates changes in hemodynamics and organ blood flow during permissive hypercapnia. Crit Care Med 24:827-834

33. Taylor DE, Gutierrez G (1996) Tonometry: a review of clinical studies. Crit Care Med 12:1007-1018
34. Van Der Linden P, Rousiu I, Deltell A et al (1995) Detection of tissue hypoxia by arteriove-nous gradient for PCO2 and pH in anesthetized dogs during progressive hemorrhage. Anesth Analg 80:269-275
35. Vallet B, Teboul JL, Coin S et al (2000) Venoarterial CO2 difference during regional ischemic or hypoxic hypoxia. J Appl Physiol 89:1317-1321
36. Schlichtig R, Bowles SA (1994) Distinguishing between aerobic and anaerobic appearance of dissolved CO2 in intestine during low flow. J Appl Physiol 76:2443-2451
37. Neviere R, Chagnon JL, Teboul JL et al (2002) Small intestine intramucosal PCO2 and mi-crovascular blood during hypoxic and ischemic hypoxia. Crit Care Med , 30:379-384
38. Dubin A, Murias G, Esterissoro E et al (2003) Intramucosal-arterial PCO2 gap fails to reflect intestinal dysoxia in hypoxic hypoxia. Crit Care Med 6:514-520
39. Gutierrez G (2004) A mathematical Model of tissue-blood CO2 exchange during hypoxia. Am J Resp Crit Care Med 169:525-530
40. Nuckton TJ, Alonsoj A, Kellet RH et al (2002) Pulmonary dead-space fraction as a risk fac-tor for death in ARDS. NJM 346:1281-1286
41. Hickling KG, Henderson SJ, Jackson R (1990) Low mortality associated with low volume pressure limited ventilation with permissive hypercapnia in severe ARDS. Int Care Med 16:372-377
42. Amato MBP, Barbas CSV, Medeiros DP et al (1995) Beneficial effects of the open lung ap-proach with low distending pressure in ARDS: a prospective randomized study on mechani-cal ventilation. Am J Resp Crit Care Med 152:1835-1846
43. Carvalho CBR, Barbas CSV, Medeiros DM et al (1997) Temporal hemodynamic effects of permissive hypercapnia associated with ideal PEEP. Am J Resp Crit Care Med 156:1458-1466
44. Carvalho CBR, Barbas CSV, Medeiros DM et al (1998) Effect of protective-ventilation strat-egy on mortality in the ARDS. N Engl J Med 338:347-354

Are We Sure We Are Using Drugs Correctly in Critical Patients?

8

Biagio Allaria

8.1 Introduction

In this chapter the words 'pharmacokinetic' and 'pharmacodynamic' will be used a number of times. It is important to explain that pharmacokinetics is the study of the absorption, distribution, metabolism and elimination of a drug and therefore allows us to predict plasma concentrations. Pharmacodynamics is the next step and is an analysis of the drug's efficacy.

The relationship between pharmacokinetics and pharmacodynamics must be optimised in order to fully enjoy the positive effects of a drug whilst minimising its toxic effects. Unfortunately the recommended doses we administer are usually determined by studying pharmacokinetics and pharmacodynamics in healthy volunteers.

But it is not that simple in intensive care. The constant variability in the status of critical patients means that pharmacokinetics and pharmacodynamics are always changing, and we must try to understand this problem in order to administer drugs appropriately. We are not talking about combination treatment, which is the norm in intensive care and an approach that is often adopted without taking drug interactions into account or understanding that many of the drugs we use are metabolised by cytochrome CYP450 isoenzymes (the CYP450 system) and that this system can be either inhibited or stimulated depending on the clinical situation.

In this chapter we shall attempt to shed light on typical clinical situations encountered in ICUs that modify the pharmacokinetics and pharmacodynamics of drugs that interfere with the CYP450 system.

B. Allaria (✉)
Past Director of Critical Care Department
Istituto Nazionale per lo Studio e la Cura dei Tumori - National Cancer Institute, Milan, Italy
e-mail: biagio.allaria@tiscali.it

Biagio Allaria (ed.), *Practical Issues in Anesthesia and Intensive Care*
© Springer-Verlag Italia 2012

8.2   Pharmacokinetic Changes: Absorption, Distribution, Metabolism and Elimination of Drugs in ICU

8.2.1   Absorption

Drugs used in ICUs are chiefly administered via the intravenous route. There is therefore little experience with the problem of variability in absorption via other routes. It is not rare, however, for patients to be treated orally, especially in the recovery phase, sometimes to enable transfer to non-specialist wards for treatment for which continuous monitoring is less of a priority or for equipment such as infusion pumps which are often insufficient outside intensive care. The amount of the drug that enters the circulation compared to the amount administered varies greatly in such cases and differ from what we usually predict following intravenous use. If we say that the bioavailability of an intravenously administered drug is 100%, the bioavailability of an extravenous drug would be a variable percentage based not only on clinical conditions but also the patient's individual characteristics.

It would be useful if extravenous use (intramuscular, subcutaneous, transcutaneous, and oral) was followed up carefully by evaluating the effect from a clinical perspective – for example, in the case of furosemide. Switching from intravenous infusions to oral treatment leads greater interindividual variability in absorption, ranging from 80% to 10%. This means that to achieve the same diuretic effect with a single dose, we would have to administer anything from 25 mg to 200 mg.

It is useful to know that another loop diuretic, torasemide, is absorbed more uniformly and that the effect of one 10 mg tablet is much easier to predict.

Another example is the absorption of subcutaneously administered low-weight molecular heparins. It is clear that if a patient has considerable cutaneous vasoconstriction (i.e. those with shock and/or treated with noradrenaline, or with serious hypovolaemia, etc.) subcutaneous absorption of the drug will be problematic and it will be useful to check aPTT more often to test efficacy. It should not come as a surprise when the expected effect is not obtained if in similar patients we use drugs with transcutaneous absorption such as clonidine and nitrate derivates.

One drug that should not longer be used subcutaneously in critical patients due to its unreliable absorption is insulin; it should always be administered intravenously in intensive care.

With transcutaneous absorption it should always be remembered that a patient's hydration status also influences the efficacy of this route of administration. In normal conditions there is partial corneum hydration (containing 7% water); this results in a ten-fold increase in drug absorption [1]. Considerable dehydration, albeit rare in critical patients, therefore makes the percutaneous route unreliable for the administration of drugs such as nitroglycerin, clonidine and analgesics.

When addressing the subject of absorption in critical patients, it is often forgotten that there are two particularly useful routes besides the oral, transcutaneous, subcutaneous, intramuscular, rectal and intravenous routes when rapid venous access is not possible: intraosseous and tracheal.

The intraosseous absorption of drugs is comparable to central venous absorption [2]. Rapid absorption is possible thanks to the venous plexus, which is reached via this route and which is not collapsible. The proximal section of the tibia is the best site for intraosseous access, which can be facilitated by commercially available kits.

When urgent resuscitation is required, i.e. when the venous route is not readily available, the intraosseous route is recommended by the American Heart Association (AHA). Only as a second resort does the AHA recommend the tracheal route, which enables decent absorption of substances with the acronym NAVEL (naloxone, atropine, vasopressin, epinephrine and lidocaine).

The absorption rate via this route is not certain, but in any case the dose required to obtain the same therapeutic effect that can be achieved via the venous route is two to two-and-a-half times he recommendation for the intravenous route. The drug is diluted in 5 mL to 10 mL of water or a saline solution, and after administration it enters the airways with repeated manual ventilation. Some authors maintain that the dilution of substances in water improves absorption compared to dilution in a saline solution.

8.2.2 Distribution

This is the process by which the drug leaves the circulation and enters the interstitium (extracellular space) and cells (intracellular space).

The extent of distribution of a drug is commonly called the "volume of distribution", a pharmacokinetic parameter consisting of the ratio between the amount of the drug in the body and the amount in the blood or plasma. Therefore, a drug with a high volume of distribution is one that is widely distributed in the body, whereas a drug with a low volume of distribution is one that tends to remain in the blood or plasma. The volume of distribution is influenced by a large number of factors such as pH, cardiac output, plasma protein binding, peripheral blood flow and vascular permeability, all of which can considerably affect distribution of the drug to tissues in critical patients.

We shall see how each of these factors can influence the distribution of drugs and consequently their efficacy.

Changes in pH

Drugs are mostly weak acids or weak alkalis and their ionisation state depends on the medium around them. Considering that drugs in an ionised state are less lipophile and therefore have trouble crossing cell membranes with a phospholipid bilayer and that, as we have already said, the pH of the medium around the drug is determined by its ionisation status, one can see how changes in pH, which are common in critical patients, can affect the volume of distribution.

There is an equation that compares the pH of the drug medium and its pK_a (acid dissociation constant), which makes it possible to calculate the percentage of the drug that is ionised and non-ionised.

We cannot claim that in daily practice we can accurately predict the volume of distribution of the drugs we use based on their pK_a and patients' pH, but we do know that wide-ranging variations in patients' pH can affect efficacy.

Plasma Protein Binding

Many drugs are characterised by non-specific plasma protein binding and tissular protein binding, especially with albumin in the case of acidic drugs and with alpha-1-acid glycoprotein in the case of alkaline drugs. The bound or non-bound fractions are in equilibrium and the amount of the bound drug depends on its affinity for proteins and on the capacity for protein binding. Only the non-bound fraction can penetrate cell membranes and is thus available for distribution, metabolism and subsequent elimination; it is therefore this fraction that interacts with specific receptors and explains the pharmacological and toxicological effects [3].

Since critical patients (most strikingly those with sepsis) often have changes in endothelial permeability with the consequent movement of proteins into the extravasal space, the result is that the protein-bound fraction largely enters this space, reaching concentrations that are higher than those in the plasma [4].

Moreover, decreased albumin and increased alphas-1-acid glycoprotein in intensive care patients is anything but rare: therefore in the case of acidic drugs that are bound to albumin, such as diazepam, the non-bound fraction increases and therefore has a greater effect whilst with alkaline drugs, such as meperidine, an increase in the protein-bound fraction can be predicted and, along with it, less efficacy.

In specific situations, high doses of a drug can completely saturate plasma protein binding sites, sharply increase the non-bound fraction and consequently the effect.

In any case it is useful to know that the effect of many drugs used in ICUs can change based on protein binding. Benet and Homer [5] have listed twenty-five such drugs, including fentanyl, propofol, midazolam, haloperidol and diltiazem, which are frequently used in our domain.

Passage of the Drug Into Interstitial Fluids and Cavities

When active substances come into contact with peripheral tissues, they usually reach the site where they are activated, but in certain situations in which some of the fluid, for a number of different reasons, is diverted from the circulation to the interstitium (oedema) or cavities (ascites, pleural effusion, pericardial effusion, etc.), they are diluted in what is commonly called the 'third space'.

Hydrophilic drugs such as aminoglycosides are dispersed in the third space, reducing the possibility of achieving sufficient concentrations at sites where they are activated. The volume of distribution of these drugs therefore increases in such situations and their efficacy is simultaneously reduced. Examples include oedemas in patients with sepsis, heart disease, cirrhosis, multiple trauma and fluid overloading. These are all situations in which effective drug concentrations and therefore efficacy are decreased.

This is particularly evident with antibiotics that have 'concentration-dependent' efficacy because in such situations they do not reach sufficient concentrations. Aminoglycosides are a classic example. It has been well documented that such deficiencies are due to the increase in the volume of distribution and the consequent reduction in plasma concentrations.

These situations are highly problematic since, on the one hand, it is necessary to raise doses to reach effective concentrations, but on the other hand concentration-dependent antibiotics such as aminoglycosides can cause renal damage, especially in patients with sepsis and serious trauma if their renal supply is often already compromised; such patients are therefore particularly susceptible to other negative factors that can later compromise renal supply.

In such cases there is no magic formula but it is essential to understand the problem and to increase renal function tests and check plasma drug concentrations.

8.2.3 Metabolism

In critical patients liver impairment is very common, with some authors stating that it occurs in 54% of patients. Since the liver is the main site of drug metabolism it is clear that impairment will affect plasma concentrations [7].

Liver impairment affecting drug metabolism in critical patients is mainly caused by changes to perfusion. In such cases, hepatic flow varies greatly and is linked not only to the course of the basic disease but also to the use of drugs such as alpha-agonists (phenylephrine, noradrenaline, vasopressin) that reduce it [8] and others, such as nitroglycerin, that increase it. De Baker [9] has demonstrated variations in hepatic flow with normal cardiac output resulting from the use of vasoactive drugs.

Besides the use of drugs, the basic disease can reduce hepatic flow, especially serious acute hypovolaemia, cardiac insufficiency and mechanical ventilation that can cause hepatic hypoperfusion. In all these situations impaired metabolism and therefore an increase in plasma concentrations can be expected.

Large amounts of various drugs administered venously in intensive care are extracted from the liver (extraction quotient > 0.7), and plasma concentrations are therefore particularly affected by decreased organ perfusion, especially with beta-blockers, morphine, midazolam and lidocaine.

The liver's metabolic activity mainly involves converting drugs into metabolites that are more soluble in water and may or may not be pharmacologically active.

Most of these processes (called 'phase I liver metabolism') are possible thanks to the presence of CYP450 isoenzymes, which we shall discuss in more detail below. The next step ('phase II') may occur without mediation of the CYP450 system and involves the conjugation of 'phase I' products with endogenous molecules such as glucuronic acid and glutathione. During phase

II, components become even more soluble and therefore easy to eliminate [10]. Both 'phase I' and 'phase II' processes are, as we have said, often changed by hepatic hypoperfusion.

8.2.4 Elimination

A large number of drugs are eliminated via the kidneys and, in particular, by means of glomerular filtration, although there are some that are actively eliminated independently of this process.

It is obvious that in patients with reduced glomerular filtration (with a resulting increase in creatininaemia) the elimination of many drugs or their catabolites may be compromised. This leads to higher plasma concentrations that may cause toxicity. A classic example of this is digoxin, the dosage of which is adjusted to each individual patient based on creatinine clearance.

Less known is the fact that at times in critical patients there may be an increase in glomerular filtration and therefore of creatinine clearance with increased cardiac output. This is possible in patients with sepsis [11], burns [12] or brain injury [13]. In such cases the clearance of hydrophilic drugs may increase, thereby reducing plasma concentrations. These patients are the same ones in whom the renal reserve is often reduced and increased plasma concentrations are most often expected. It is worth remembering this when regularly checking the creatinine clearance not only of patients with low supply (which we do routinely) but also of those with above-normal supply.

Some considerations are required for the elimination of drugs in elderly patients. In such cases the creatininaemia guide for predicting the efficiency of renal drug elimination may be wrong. In fact, a reduction in the muscular mass of elderly patients accompanies a fall in the production of creatinine, the plasma concentration of which may appear normal even in those with moderate renal insufficiency. Moreover, even in patients who do not have kidney disease creatinine clearance is usually reduced in elderly patients by 30% to 50%. When administered drugs that are eliminated via the kidneys to elderly patients it is entirely advisable not to limit oneself to creatininaemia tests but also to control creatinine clearance.

8.3 Pharmacodynamic Changes

So far we have discussed how the absorption, distribution, metabolism and elimination of drugs are influenced in particular situations that may affect critical patients and therefore, in other words, how critical situations affect the plasma concentrations of drugs. However, in addition to the plasma concentrations, the response to the drug is also affected in various clinical situations.

In critical patients, besides changes to pharmacokinetic properties, there are changes in pharmacodynamics, if by pharmacodynamics we mean the existing relationship between plasma concentrations of a drug and the pharmacological response.

An example of this is the tolerance to drugs that are used in patients with sepsis and burns [14], probably due to reduced affinity of receptors for the drugs or for changes in the intrinsic activity of receptors.

It is also necessary to take into account the fact that most drugs have their own activity in tissues and that therefore it is not plasma concentrations that count so much as tissue concentrations. Measuring the tissue concentrations of drugs is still a taboo in current clinical practice but they have been controlled using microdialysis with surprising and interesting results. For example, Zeitlinger [15] used microdialysis to measure ciprofloxacin concentrations in the muscular interstitial fluid in patients with sepsis. The concentrations did not enable drug efficacy even though plasma levels fully thought of as therapeutic. We should therefore conclude that, at least for this antibiotic, we can expect little efficacy in the muscles in patients with sepsis when usual doses are administered.

Fortunately for some drugs used in intensive care the dosage can be individualised to achieve the desired effect. This is possible for those drugs that have a rapid onset and a short duration of action, such as vasoactive drugs. In such cases, prior understanding of their behaviour in various clinical situations may be useful but is not fundamental.

For other drugs, particularly those distributed exclusively in extracellular spaces, the response is barely predictable in our patients, who demonstrate wide-ranging variability in flow and the volume of fluid in these spaces.

However, even with vasoactive drugs, the problem is not resolved with strict determination of effective doses but it is necessary to be aware of the collateral effects, which can be very severe. We shall mention just one vasoactive drug that, if it is not used entirely correctly, can cause a number of problems: nitroprusside. Hypertensive crises are anything but rare in operating rooms and ICUs and nitroprusside is one of the most effective hypotensive drugs with a venous and arterial vasodilatory effect thanks to an NO-mediated mechanism. This drug has a rapid onset and a relatively short duration of activity, and its dosage can therefore be titrated based on patient response. However, during long-term treatment nitroprusside metabolism leads to the formation of cyanide ions that bind to haemoglobin, forming cyanohaemoglobin. These ions also bind with cytochrome oxidase. The organs that suffer the most damage from this are the heart and brain. The appearance of changes in the patient's mental status, cardiovascular instability with severe arrhythmia, metabolic acidosis and, in more serious cases, seizures and coma, are the effects of this type of intoxication. Moreover, nitroprusside, a potent venous vasodilator, can cause a considerable drop in preload and thus in supply in ventilated patients, as well as tachycardia, coronary steal and increased shunt fraction due to the release of hypoxic vasoconstriction.

With all these problems it is important when choosing treatment of hypertensive crises not to forget that there are less problematic drugs that can achieve the desired effect, such as clonidine, calcium antagonists, alpha-blockers, beta-blockers, labetalol and esmolol [16]. If nitroprusside is chosen, it is best not to administer more than 8 µg/kg/min every 1-3 hours.

We cannot close this discussion without considering the pharmacodynamic changes that result from drug interactions. This is too often underestimated and, in the event of unusual responses to multiple drug treatment, drug interactions would always be part of a differential diagnosis.

There are easily consultable electronic instruments that enable the possibility of interactions between the drugs we use to be checked. One of these, called MIMN, from the Mario Negri Pharmacological Research Institute in Milan, is easily to consult and certainly an asset in ICUs where drug treatment is the norm. Here we cannot summarise the numerous drug interactions that are possible, but we can mention pharmacokinetic interactions that reduce drug availability at target sites and those that increase it.

Pharmacokinetic Interactions That Reduce Drug Availability at 'Target Sites'

One of these interactions occurs in the gastrointestinal system where some drug combinations reduce absorption. For example, since oral ketoconazole is dissolved and absorbed only in acidic media, the use of H_2-receptor antagonists (such as ranitidine) or a proton pump inhibitor (such as omeprazole) prevents sufficient absorption.

The expression of some genes responsible for drug elimination, particularly CYP3A and MDRI, can be markedly higher for certain drugs such as rifampicin, carbamazepine, phenytoin and other substances such as tobacco smoke and alcohol. Under the effect of these drugs and substances, important drugs such as verapamil, warfarin, ketoconazole, cyclosporin, dexamethasone, methylprednisolone and metronidazole are more rapidly metabolised. We therefore expect less efficacy with these drugs in patients who drink, smoke or concomitantly use rifampicin, phenytoin or carbamazepine.

It is useful to remember the contrasting aspect of this problem: a person who drinks and smokes a lot but who stops these habits during long-term treatment with oral anticoagulants and who has a satisfactory INR can expect a sudden increase in INR, which would be unforeseeable and inexplicable to someone who does not understand these concepts.

Pharmacokinetic Interactions That Increase Drug Availability at 'Target Sites'

Some drugs have a potent inhibiting action on oxidative metabolism that is the basis for the break-down of other drugs. This is true for cimetidine (but not of any other H_2-receptor antagonists), which is a potent inhibitor of the oxidative metabolism of warfarin, theophylline, nifedipine, phenytoin and lidocaine. Combined use of cimetidine and these drugs may cause serious damage.

Above we saw how the expression of the gene CYP3A decreased the effect of many drugs. On the other hand, depression of this gene increases plasma levels. Thus, some drugs that depress the expression of the gene CYP3A, such as fluconazole, ketoconazole, erythromycin, clarithromycin, diltiazem, verapamil and nicardipine (all of which are widely used in intensive care) can, by inhibiting CYP3A, lead to toxic concentrations of cyclosporin, and even very common drugs such as statins can increase the likelihood of myopathy.

It should be emphasised that, beyond the mechanisms described, there are drug interactions that also cause serious adverse effects. For example, it is known that small doses of aspirin do not affect the INR of patients treated with warfarin, but increase the risk of haemorrhage due to their platelet anti-aggregant effect. Nor do NSAIDS increase the INR of patients treated with warfarin, but triple the possibility of gastric haemorrhage due to the harmful effect they have on mucosa. NSAIDs always antagonise the antihypertensive effects of beta-blockers, diuretics, ACE inhibitors and other drugs.

Drugs that prolong the QT interval most often lead to torsades de pointes when used concomitantly with diuretics that cause potassium depletion. The use of potassium salts often causes possibly dangerous hyperpotassaemia if administered with ACE inhibitors, spironolactone, amiloride and triamterene.

The combined use in ICUs of curare-like agents, aminoglycosides and corticosteroids increases the risk of serious myopathy, i.e. so-called critical illness myopathy (CIM).

Lorazepam, which is used for continuous infusions in ICUs, can cause possibly serious metabolic acidosis due to a molecule in it that acts as a carrier: propylene glycol. This substance is usually metabolised in the liver and eliminated unchanged in the urine. In patients with renal and hepatic impairment, which is common in intensive care, propylene glycol accumulates, causing hyperosmolar metabolic acidosis. This is exacerbated in combination with other drugs containing propylene glycol, such as trimethoprim-sulfamethoxazole, nitroglycerin and phenytoin. There may be an endless number of examples, but we have only mentioned a few in order to encourage anaesthetists and providers of resuscitation to tackle the subject of drug interactions more systematically.

8.3.1 CYP450 and Interactions with CYP450-Mediated Drugs in Intensive Care

We have already mentioned some drug interactions that are mediated by the CYP450 system, but this system is the basis of metabolism for most drugs used in intensive care and is worth addressing separately.

In the CYP450 family there are some enzymes responsible for drug metabolism: CYP3A4, CYP2C9, CYP219, CYP2D6, CYP1A2. They are the basis for important interactions between problematic drugs often used in ICUs.

Drug Interactions Mediated by CYP3A4
CYP3A4 is possibly the most important enzyme involved in drug metabolism. It accounts for 50% of all enzymes in the CYP450 family and manages the bio-oxidative transformation of at least 50% of drugs that are metabolised by means of an oxidative mechanism.

CYP3A4 is expressed in both the liver and the intestinal epithelium and therefore its inhibition or induction may occur at either of these sites, affecting the absorption and hepatic break-down of drugs. If a drug is administered orally, CYP3A4 is induced, less of the drug is absorbed and, when it reaches the liver, it is more rapidly metabolised. The result is that drug bioavailability is reduced, leading to low efficacy.

Rifampicin, phenytoin, carbamazepine and phenobarbital are potent CYP3A4 inducers.

Conversely, if CYP3A4 is inhibited, a greater amount of the drug is absorbed in the intestines and less is metabolised by the liver. Bioavailability is thus increased, with the possibility of reaching toxic plasma concentrations. Antifungal agents (azoles), calcium antagonists and macrolides (erythromycin and clarithromycin) can inhibit CYP3A4.

We have seen which drugs act on CYP3A4 and therefore have insufficient plasma levels when induced, or potentially toxic plasma levels when inhibited. They are drugs frequently used in intensive care: midazolam, cyclosporin, tacrolimus, fentanyl (not remifentanil) and methylprednisolone.

In particular there are studies that show a complete loss of effect for midazolam when used concomitantly with potential CYP3A4 inducers such as phenytoin and rifampicin [17, 18] and increased plasma levels reaching 300% when used with potent CYP3A4 inhibitors such as fluconazole in continuous infusions, with excessive sedation leading to coma.

Specifically, the combination of fluconazole with cyclosporin, which is often used after transplants, requires frequent plasma concentration controls for cyclosporin, which may reach toxic levels. Similarly, but in an opposite way, plasma cyclosporin levels are to be controlled if rifampicin is also administered: in this case the cyclosporin dosage may be insufficient and the transplanted organ may be rejected.

Drug Interactions Mediated by CYP2C9 and CYP2C19

These two enzymes are important in the absorption and metabolism of phenytoin. When combined with an infusion of a potent inhibitor of both these enzymes, such as fluconazole, phenytoin reaches toxic levels (> 25 mg/dL), causing mental confusion, respiratory depression and coma.

Phenytoin itself is an inducer of these enzymes and therefore reduces plasma fluconazole levels when used simultaneously. Using these two drugs together leads to toxic phenytoin concentrations and renders fluconazole ineffective.

Another drug greatly affected by CYP2C9 is warfarin. Although it is now known that genetic variations in CYP2C9 are the basis of wide variability in patients' response to warfarin, in this case too CYP2C9 inhibitors such as fluconazole potentiate the effect of warfarin whilst inducers such as rifampicin have the opposite effect.

Drug Interactions Mediated by CYP2D6

CYP2D6 was the first example of genetic polymorphism. There are patients, so-called fast metabolisers (1-2% of the population) who have exacerbated activity for this enzyme and rapidly break down drugs such as opioids, beta-blockers and SSRIs. Other patients are so-called slow metabolisers, in whom plasma concentrations of these drugs reach higher levels than predicted with usual doses (5-10% of the population).

Inducers of CYP2D6 have not been described, while inhibitors such as quinidine, haloperidol, paroxetine and fluoxetine are known. With the concomitant administration of haloperidol and beta-blockers potentiation of the effect of beta-blockers can be expected, with bradycardia and unforeseeable hypotension if the problem is not recognised.

8.4   Conclusion

The ongoing variability in clinical conditions for critical patients results in frequent variation in the pharmacokinetics and pharmacodynamics of the main drugs used. The use of drugs is almost always vital in intensive care and multiple drugs are almost always used.

The correct use of drugs in critical patients is anything but straightforward. It is necessary to know the pharmacokinetic properties in normal conditions for the substances that are to be used, but there are simple ways in which to do this since there are numerous publications, such as that by Power [19], that illustrate the pharmacokinetic properties of the main drugs used in intensive care. Power's work is very useful as it describes the pharmacokinetics of most drugs used in critical patients.

Yet this only the first step, since, as we have said in this chapter, critical patients have trouble absorbing drugs (when they are not administered venously), as well as with distribution, metabolism and elimination, which are not always recognised in intensive care, whilst the problem of relativising these changes in terms of how they affect plasma drug concentrations and subsequently drug efficacy is not easy to identify by intensive care physicians. The aim of this chapter is to assist intensive care physicians to understand these relationships by providing numerous practical examples that contain important advice on the correct use of many drugs.

The argument is, however, very complex and deserves further discussion. We would like to recommend the excellent work published by Roncher in 2006 [20] for those who would like to study the issue further, since it comprehensively covers the steps we have discussed in this chapter and provides useful practical advice.

In general the literature agrees on the following points:
- we should understand the basic pharmacokinetic and pharmacodynamic properties of each of the active substances we use;

- we should know the effects that various clinical situations have on the absorption, distribution, metabolism and elimination of drugs;
- we should consider drug interactions when administering concomitant treatment;
- in specific situations such as critical patients we should, when possible, adjust dosages according to patient response and, when this is not possible, control plasma drug concentrations more frequently.

This chapter, unfortunately, is not able to solve all these problems (as with other publications on the subject), but it is an attempt for more a rational treatment approach in critical patients.

Bibliography

1. Galli CL, Corsini E (2004) Tossicologia, Piccin, Padova
2. Bershad EM et al (2007) Know the alternate routes for administration of cardiopulmonary re-suscitation medication. Avoiding common ICU errors. Walters Kluwer/ Lippincott Williams and Wilkins, Philadelphia
3. Herve F et al (1994) Drug binding in plasma. A summary of recent trends in the study of drug and hormone binding. Clin Pharmacokinet 26:44-58
4. Lin X et al (2009) Optimizing drug dosing in ICU. In: Vincent JL, Yearbook of Intensive care and emergency medicine, Springer, Heidelberg
5. Benet LZ, Hoener AA (2002) Changes in plasma protein binding have little clinical relevance. Clin Pharmacol Ther 71:115-121
6. Reaand RS, Capitano B (2007) Optimizing use of aminoglycosides in the critically ill. Semin CritCare Med 28:596-603
7. Power BM et al (1998) Pharmacokinetics of drugs used in critically ill adults. Clin Pharma-cokinetic 34:25-56
8. Obritsch MD et al (2004) The role of vasopressin in vasodilatory septic shock. Pharma-cotherapy 24:1050-1063
9. De Backer D et al (2003) Effect of dopamine, norepinephrine and epinephrine on the splanch-nic circulation in septic shock: which is best? Crit Care Med 31:1659-1667
10. Spriet I, Meersseman N (2009) Relevant CYP450 mediated drug interactions in the ICU. In: Vincent JL, Yearbook of intensive care and emergency medicine, pp 870-877. Springer, Hei-delberg Springer
11. Kumar A et al (2006) Duration of hypotension before initiation of effective antimicrobial therapy in the critical determinant of survival in human septic shock. Crit Care Med 34:1589-1596
12. Weinbreu MJ (1999) Pharmacokinetics of antibiotic in burn patients. J Antimicrobial Chemio-ther 44:319-327
13. Lipman J et al (2003) Cefepine vs. cefpizone: the importance of creatinine clearance. Anesth Analg 97:1149-1154
14. Tschida SJ et al (1995) Atracurium resistance in critically ill patients. Pharmacotherapy 15:533-553
15. Zeitlinger MA et al (2003) Relevance of soft tissue penetration by levofloxacin for target site bacterial killing in patients with sepsis. Antimicrob Agents Chemother 47:3548-3553
16. Bravos ED (2007) The alert for the development of cyanide toxicity when administering ni-troprusside. In: Marcucci et al, Avoiding common ICU errors, p 48. Kluwer/Lippincott, Philadelphia

17. Finch CK et al (2002) Rifampin and rifabutin drug interactions. An update. Arch Int Med 162:985-992
18. Perucca E (2005) Clinically relevant drug interaction with antiepileptic drugs. Brit J Clin Pharmacol 61:246-255
19. Powe BM et al (1998) Pharmacokinetics of drugs used in critically ill adults. Clin Pharmacokinetic 34: 25-56
20. Boucher BA et al (2006) Pharmacokinetics changes in critically illness. Crit Care Clin 22:255-271

The Problem of Decontamination of the Digestive Tract and Gastric Acid Suppression in Intensive Care

9

Biagio Allaria

9.1 Introduction

Both therapeutic strategies mentioned in the title of this chapter have an important role in the management of critical patients.

The first – decontamination of the digestive tract – aims to reduce the incidence of pneumonia; the second – gastric acid suppression – seeks to prevent stress ulcers and consequently gastrointestinal haemorrhage. Yet there is still plenty of confusion surrounding them.

Decontamination of the digestive tract, for example, is not included in guidelines for the prevention of pneumonia [1], but there are numerous studies that support it and the best way to implement it is still a subject of debate. It is still unclear whether selective decontamination of the digestive tract (SDD) [2, 3] or selective oropharyngeal decontamination (SOD) is the best approach [4, 5].

In terms of suppressing the secretion of acid in the stomach, there is still a debate about the best drugs to use: H_2-receptor antagonists (ranitidine, famotidine, etc.) or proton pump inhibitors (PPIs) such as omeprazole and lansoprazole, or whether it is not merely best to protect gastric mucosa with sucralfate.

Furthermore, an increase in the incidence of pneumonia has repeatedly been described in patients in whom gastric acid is suppressed, and this type of adverse effect is precisely what we want to reduce with SDD or SOD.

These two therapeutic strategies, even with a positive value in the prevention of complications in intensive care, would seem to have the opposite effect in the prevention of pneumonia.

B. Allaria (✉)
Past Director of Critical Care Department
Istituto Nazionale per lo Studio e la Cura dei Tumori - National Cancer Institute, Milan, Italy
e-mail: biagio.allaria@tiscali.it

In this chapter we shall discuss decontamination of the digestive tract and gastric acid suppression separately and we shall attempt to understand whether it is appropriate for these two strategies to be associated in the management of critical patients.

9.2   Decontamination of the Digestive Tract

The prevention of infections, especially in the respiratory apparatus, is a cornerstone of the management of critical patients, since infections play a significant role in terms of mortality, morbidity, duration of hospitalisation and costs [6].

SDD and SOD have yielded satisfactory results in the prevention of respiratory infections.

SDD involves the prevention and colonisation of Gram-negative microorganisms, *Staphylococcus aureus* and yeasts using non-absorbable antimicrobial agents in the oropharynx and the gastrointestinal tract, as well as the systemic use of cephalosporin for four days in order to eliminate a possible bacterial component in the respiratory apparatus, which results in the avoidance of antibiotics that could damage anaerobic intestinal flora, whether generally or locally [7].

There is considerable agreement about the possibility of reducing the incidence of infections with SDD, but most studies do not include enough subjects to demonstrate definite efficacy in reducing mortality. Yet three studies are available from single study centres [2, 3, 8] as well as a meta-analysis [9] that seem to show that SDD is effective in lowering mortality rates.

SOD (using topical oropharyngeal administration of antibiotics alone) has been proposed as an alternative to SDD for the prevention of pneumonia associated with the use of respiratory devices (ventilator-associated pneumonia, VAP) [4, 5]. There is considerable agreement on the possibility that oropharyngeal bacterial colonisation plays a role in VAP) [10, 11]. There is sufficient evidence regarding the efficacy of SOD too, which seems to demonstrate as much efficacy as SDD in preventing VAP [12, 13], but until January 2009, when Smet et al. [15] published a study in 5,939 patients, there were no large-scale studies in numerous subjects that address SDD, SOD and conventional treatment without decontamination. Below we shall discuss this study in further detail.

In the absence of any studies of this type, the lack of certainty, especially regarding the possibility of decontamination of the digestive tract, may result in the selection of antibiotic-resistant pathogens, meaning that this procedure is not one of the strategies recommended in the international guidelines on VAP prevention published in 2005 [14].

The SDD procedure used in Smet's study, which is identical to that employed by de Jounge in 2003 [2], is based on the intravenous administration of cefotaxime during the first four days of application in the oropharynx and stomach of a paste composed of tobramycin, polymyxin and amphoteracin B, according to the following list:

- Paste applied to oropharyngeal cavity four times per day (0.5 g), containing: 2% polymyxin, 2% tobramycin, 2% amphotericin B
- Solution inserted into gastric catheter containing: 100 mg polymyxin E, 80 mg tobramycin, 500 mg amphotericin B
- In patients having undergone tracheotomy, the paste is applied to the oropharynx around the tracheostomy four times per day
- In patients having undergone colostomy, suppositories are also used four times per day containing: 42 mg amphotericin B, 42 mg polymyxin E, 64 mg, tobramycin
- In all patients, 1 g to 4 g cefotaxime is administered for the first four days
- Enteral nourishment is initiated as soon as possible

The use of antibiotics with anaerobic activity such as amoxicillin, amoxicillin + clavulanic acid and carbapenems was avoided as much as possible. In the same study SOD was based on the oropharyngeal application of the same paste as was used for SDD. In this case, however, there were no restrictions on the systemic use of antibiotics.

The effects of the decontamination strategy on mortality are encouraging as there was a 13% reduction with SDD and 11% with SOD compared to the control group without decontamination. These results took into account the fact that, although the authors had done what they could to obtain homogeneous groups of patients, the groups treated with SDD and SOD were older, had a higher Apache II score, a lower incidence of surgical causes for admission and a longer duration of mechanical ventilation compared to the control group. Patients treated with decontamination therefore had greater risk factors.

The average proportion of episodes of bacteriaemia during hospitalisation was lower in the SDD group (6.5%) and SOD group (4.3%) than the control group (9.3%), but of particular interest was the reduction in the incidence of bacteriaemia caused by *Staphylococcus aureus* and Gram-negative microorganisms, which was halved.

The study also assessed the degree of eradication of Gram-negative bacteria from the intestinal and respiratory tracts that were judged satisfactory either with SDD or SOD. Both decontamination strategies helped to lower the incidence of oropharyngeal and intestinal colonisation by Gram-negative antibiotic-resistant microorganisms compared to the control group and this seems to confirm what had already been stated, namely that SDD is not associated with increased selection of antibiotic-resistant microorganisms nor the induction of antibiotic resistance, at least in media that are not characterised by high levels of multiresistant Gram-negative microorganisms in the blood. Yet the previous assertion that in media in which multiresistant Gram-negative fungi and methicillin-resistant *Staphylococcus aureus* (MRSA) are frequent, SDD can increase the selection of these pathogens, is still true [16, 17, 18].

This study, which, as we said before, is to be considered fundamental, therefore concludes that, since SDD and SOD have similar results in terms of mortality and the incidence of bacteriaemia, it seems reasonable to opt for SOD in future as it is easier to implement, cheaper (1 USD per day compared to 12 USD for SDD), does not require cephalosporin administration for four days, and allows for the use of antibiotics such as amoxicillin and carbapenems.

Since the simplified method of decontamination (SOD) seems to have the same effect at the more complex method (SDD), it may be useful to consider a simplified procedure at a later point that substitutes the multiple-antibiotic paste with an antiseptic agent such as chlorhexidine, especially in media characterised by a high level of antibiotic resistance.

9.2.1　SOD with Chlorhexidine

Considering the large amount of equivalence between SDD and SOD in the prevention of infections in intensive care and the lower cost, the lower use and the absence of accompanying antibiotic in SOD, it is clear that SOD is the strategy of choice if digestive decontamination is to be a routine procedure.

Yet the procedure would be simpler still if in place of the multiple antibiotic paste one could use a single antiseptic solution. This appears possible, since a study by Koeman et al. published in 2006 seems to demonstrate the efficacy of chlorhexidine used in this way [19]. The authors studied three different VAP prevention protocols in 385 patients: a control group with the traditional method, a group treated with chlorhexidine and another group receiving chlorhexidine+colimycin.

The group treated with chlorhexidine+colimycin was associated with the awareness that chlorhexidine is effective against Gram-positive microorganisms, even multi-resistant microorganisms, including MRSA and vancomycin-resistant *Enterococcus* (VRE) but much less effective against Gram-negative microorganisms. This was a randomised, double-blind, placebo-controlled trial with 2% chlorhexidine in vaseline applied with a gloved finger four times per day in the mouth. The incidence of VAP was 18% in the control group and 13% in both the chlorhexidine group and chlorhexidine+colimycin group.

As expected, the group treated with chlorhexidine+colimycin showed a lower incidence of Gram-negative colonisation but, as we have seen, without influencing the incidence of VAP. It therefore seems that decontamination of the oral cavity with chlorhexidine can be advised as a useful strategy for preventing VAP, even if mortality in the reports published by Koeman was identical in the three groups. VAP reduction, however, involves a reduction in the length of hospital stay and costs.

It is therefore stated that, if it is true that SOD with three antibiotics has been shown to reduce mortality in Smet's large-scale study, it is also true that it can be seen from the statistical analysis with which the incidence of this is defined that it was correct based on risk factors in the treatment and control groups. Mortality without adjustments was similar to that of the Koeman study.

However, Koeman attempts to explain the lack of evidence for a reduction in VAP mortality in his study, pointing out that VAP mortality has wide-ranging variability in international studies, varying from 0% to 50%. The author correctly states that mortality is inversely proportional to treatment accuracy. When treatment is appropriate, mortality is low and if we were to compare the advantages of various treatments, we would need greater numbers than those included in the studies. The author shows that using antiseptic as well as common antibiotic agents such as those used in SDD and SOD incurs a lower risk of selecting microorganisms that are resistant to many of the drugs most often used in intensive care.

9.2.2 Discussion on Digestive Decontamination

When in 1994 Bouten et al. [10] published in *Chest* their study on the possible role of bacterial colonisation of the stomach, oropharynx and trachea in influencing the incidence of pneumonia in ICUs, it was clear that gastric colonisation did not have an important function in that respect. The title of their work was revealing: *"The stomach is not a source for colonization of the upper respiratory tract and pneumonia in ICU patients"*. It would appear from their study that decontamination forces were concentrated in the oropharyngeal cavity and trachea rather than the stomach.

After this study, however, the number of studies using SDD for VAP prevention increased, with decontamination of either the oropharyngeal or gastric cavities. The results are rather encouraging but it is not clear if the efficacy of the procedure was linked to gastric or oropharyngeal decontamination or both. Moreover, the possibility of non-multiple-antibiotic oropharyngeal decontamination was raised but with an antiseptic, which made the choice of strategy harder.

In 2007 Chan et al. [12] published an interesting meta-analysis of eleven trials involving a total of 3,242 patients, comparing the efficacy of oropharyngeal decontamination with antibiotics against decontamination with chlorhexidine decontamination. With all the restrictions of this type of meta-analysis it nevertheless seemed that the authors were able to confirm that, compared with the control group (without decontamination), the entire oropharyngeal decontamination group had a lower incidence of VAP but that this was almost entirely due to the results obtained with chlorhexidine.

Simpler support for oropharyngeal decontamination with antiseptic agents emerged from the study by Sierra [20] in Spanish ICUs published in *Chest* in 2005. 93% of ICUs used antiseptic agents for decontamination of the oral cavity whilst only one ICU used SDD with multiple antibiotics.

It therefore seems to be the case from the international literature and from common ICU practices that there is a preference for SOD with antiseptic agents as the strategy for decontamination of the digestive tract.

However, in several studies published there are limits to the diagnosis of VAP, which at times was carried out on the basis of microbiological and microscopic data from specimens obtained by means of BAL and/or swabs rather than with clinical and radiological data, at other times with tracheal aspiration, and sometimes with radiological and clinical data alone. The rather inaccurate diagnosis of VAP has, as one can imagine, little specificity and therefore over-estimates the incidence of VAP. This makes it difficult to compare studies from different centres with various practices and to interpret meta-analyses.

We have stressed the fact that one of the areas that can influence the choice of SOD with antiseptic agents is that this would enable the possible selection of antibiotic-resistant microorganisms to be avoided, which are often valuable in the treatment of infections in intensive care. This seems important from a the-oretical perspective but contradicts the observation of various working groups that have not found this after digestive decontamination procedures. In particu-lar, the study by Henninger [12] published in 2006 is interesting as, after five years of routine use of SDD in ICUs he did not find any selection of multi-resistant microorganisms.

Finally we can conclude that digestive decontamination is a safe and effec-tive practice and that, managed alongside an antiseptic agent such as chlorhex-idine in the oropharynx alone, it may be widely used in intensive care through-out the world.

9.3   Gastric Acid Suppression in Intensive Care in the Prophylaxis of Stress Ulcers

More than ten years ago an observational study was performed in a single day in twenty different hospitals in Italy with the purpose of understanding the number of hospitalised patients undergoing gastric acid suppression. The results were surprising: 27% of those admitted received such treatment and in 51% of cases it was inappropriate [22].

The situation appears not have changed in recent years, with the develop-ment of proton pump inhibitors (PPIs) such as omeprazole and lansoprazole. The percentage of hospitalised patients undergoing gastric acid suppression continues to increase and is now estimated to be somewhere between 40% and 70%, with at least 50% of patients beginning such therapy in hospital.

Yet there is no lack of alarms on the non-critical use of this treatment and it is thought that it is inappropriate in 70% of cases [23].

For example, more and more data are emerging in the literature on the increasing incidence of nosocomial pneumonia in patients treated with PPIs or H_2-receptor antagonists. A study published in *JAMA* in 2009 [24] in a very large number of hospitalised patients (63,878 patients) effectively demonstrat-ed that gastric acid suppression increases nosocomial pneumonia by 30%, but the fact that this adverse effect is linked particularly to PPIs and not H_2-recep-tor antagonists (ranitidine, famotidine, etc.) is of great interest. The authors even go as far as estimating that the inappropriate use of this treatment may cause 33,000 avoidable deaths every year in the United States.

Of equal interest is the finding that pneumonia in patients treated with PPIs is confirmed particularly in the first two days of treatment and that the incidence decreases over time. This pattern is exactly the opposite of what is expected if we think, as we always have, of the transfer of gastric bacteria (which by reducing acidity becomes a less hostile medium for bacteria) to the trachea and airways. If this were so, the incidence of pneumonia would increase over time with a gradual decrease in acidity that promotes gastric colonisation. In reality, a certain level of doubt has accompanied this process for some time. At the beginning of this chapter we referred to the work by Bouten that appeared in *Chest* with the title: *"The stomach is not the source for colonization of the upper respiratory tract and pneumonia in ICU patients"* [10]. In this study an accurate bi-weekly microbiological review was conducted of bacterial colonisation in the stomach, oropharynx and trachea in patients receiving mechanical ventilation, and the existing relation between colonisation and VAP episodes was studied. A convincing colonisation sequence was found in no patients from the stomach to the upper airways and this demonstrated to the authors that the stomach was not the most common bacterial source in their patients, who were all receiving H$_2$-receptor antagonists for the prevention of stress ulcers.

Already the idea that H$_2$-receptor antagonists could play a role in causing pneumonia was a matter of debate.

Therefore, for many years, H$_2$-receptor antagonists used in the prevention of stress ulcers have been regarded with less suspicion in the tricky interpretation of the causes of nosocomial pneumonia and, in particular, of those patients in ICUs receiving mechanical ventilation. Yet, as we have pointed out, this observation cannot easily be extrapolated to the wide range of drugs used in the treatment and prevention of ulcers: PPIs. For these drugs a different reality emerges, which seems to be involved in causing pneumonia yet with a potentially different mechanism from that of gastric acid suppression.

9.3.1 Can Proton Pump Inhibitors Facilitate Infections with a Diverse Mechanism for the Suppression of Gastric Acid?

The action of omeprazole, the progenitor of PPIs, blocks (H$^+$+K$^+$)-ATPase in the stomach, but this blocking action can also affect another enzyme, (Na$^+$/K$^+$)-ATPase, which plays a fundamental role in the function of natural killer (NK) cells, which themselves are important in defence mechanisms for infections. Theoretically, therefore, since omeprazole can block the (Na$^+$+K$^+$)-ATPase system in the stomach, it can also block it systemically and therefore negatively interfere with the immune system by blocking the cytotoxic action of NK cells.

The problem was already addressed fifteen years ago by Aybay, who published a study about the effect of omeprazole on NK cells [25]. In this study the author showed that omeprazole was able to block the (Na$^+$+K$^+$)-ATPase system and therefore inhibit its cytotoxic effect, but at plasma concentrations that were not reached using the drug at commonly recommended doses. This study therefore confirmed the theoretical interference of omeprazole with the immune system, but also seemed to rule out the fact that it could occur at doses usually used in clinical practice.

However, a lot of attention is still being paid to the possibility that PPIs may reduce the defence mechanism and thus facilitate infections, particularly in ICUs, and some years after Aybay's study, in 2002, Zedwitz-Liebenstein et al. [26], from the Infectious Diseases Department of the University of Vienna, published a fundamental study on the effects of omeprazole on neutrophil function. Neutrophils are the first line of defence for cells during bacterial invasions and their importance was shown by the increased incidence of infections in patients with neutropenia.

An in vitro effect that inhibited the capacity of omeprazole on neutrophils to produce the enzyme superoxide, which is significant in explaining bactericidal activity, was already shown by Wandall in 1992 [27] but the action of omeprazole on healthy volunteers was an important focus by Zedwitz-Liebenstein.

It is difficult to say how important these mechanisms are in increasing the incidence of nosocomial pneumonia during PPI treatment, but there are, as we have said, sufficient studies to enable us to take this into account.

Similar negative effects on neutrophil function were not demonstrated by H2-receptor antagonists (ranitidine, cimetidine, famotidine) in a study by Mikawa published in 1999 [32].

The negative effect of omeprazole on granulocyte function, which in many ways is undesirable due to its anti-bactericidal action, could, however, be useful in situations such as acute pancreatitis where the accumulation of neutrophils in the lungs certainly plays a role in the exacerbation of the disease. In this case omeprazole may play a minor anti-inflammatory role in the lungs.

However, to answer the question in the title of this chapter we may say that there is enough evidence to state that cases of pneumonia that are confirmed with greater incidence in patients treated with PPIs are not only (or not so much) linked to bacterial colonisation in the stomach with bacterial transfer to the airways, but to a mechanism of interference with the cell immune system.

The difference in the incidence of pneumonia between patients treated with PPIs and those treated with H2-receptor antagonists may be linked to the fact that for the latter there do not seem to be as many obvious negative effects as for PPIs.

9.3.2 Do Considerations Concerning the Existing Relationship Between Gastric Acid Suppression and Nosocomial Pneumonia Also Apply to Intensive Care Patients? Are H2-Receptor Antagonists Interchangeable with PPIs?

We have seen that the excessive and often inappropriate use of H2-receptor antagonists and PPIs in the general hospital population is now obvious. This is absolutely disproportionate to the incidence of gastric haemorrhage of approximately 1%, and these drugs should be used more selectively for patients at a higher risk such, as those with developing or existing ulcerous disease, oesophageal reflux, known gastric erosion and established coagulation disorders.

The reality in intensive care varies greatly. Even though it has been largely reduced (perhaps thanks to the drugs we have discussed), the incidence of gastric haemorrhage in critical patients is considerably higher than that of patients admitted to non-specialist wards and is between 2.8% and 6% [33]. This mainly justifies wider use of antisecretory agents in ICUs but does not prevent us from considering that even in these areas use is excessive and often inappropriate.

In any case, the first step is to understand that H_2-receptor antagonists and PPIs, even with different mechanisms of action, are at least interchangeable from an efficacy perspective. The objective of treatment with these drugs is to reach gastric pH levels of more than 4 and that the sine qua non condition of this is to reduce the risk of bleeding.

Both H_2-receptor antagonists and PPIs are able to reach this objective quickly but there is convincing literature that states that with PPIs higher pH levels can be reached. This seems to be true especially when it is necessary to inhibit secretion for longer periods since patients quickly develop tolerance to H_2-receptor antagonist, which reduces the effect on pH over time. A similar effect is not observed with PPI.

Due to their ability to produce greater and more persistent gastric alkalinisation, PPIs are most likely to create a medium that is more favourable to bacterial colonisation in the stomach, thus promoting a higher incidence of pneumonia due to transfer of microorganisms to the airways. In reality, as we have already seen, the first large-scale study on the relationship between H_2-receptor antagonists, PPIs and nosocomial pneumonia published in *JAMA* in 2009 showed a statistically higher incidence of nosocomial pneumonia in patients treated with PPIs compared to those treated with H_2-receptor antagonists. This study mainly included patients admitted to non-specialist wards and therefore no critical patients and, above all, no patients receiving mechanical ventilation. Moreover, as we have already emphasised, pneumonia was confirmed especially in the first two days of treatment with PPIs, while an increase in alkalinisation of the gastric fluid was probable on successive days. This pattern reinforced the hypothesis that PPIs facilitate pulmonary infections not by stimulating bacterial colonisation of the stomach but by negatively interfering with the function of NK cells and neutrophilic granulocytes.

Yet if this is substantially true for nosocomial pneumonia outside ICUs, it is still uncertain for critical patients receiving mechanical ventilation. Studies that compare H_2-receptor antagonists with PPIs in critical patients cannot include as many subjects as those involving patients admitted to non-specialist wards, but we can attempt to make a few interpretations.

The study by Mallow [34], for example, which appeared in *Current Surgery* in 2004 [34], was conducted in patients with multiple trauma undergoing mechanical ventilation and found no differences in the incidence of VAP between the two patient groups, those treated with H_2-receptor antagonists and those treated with PPIs. The study was of particular interest in disregarding the importance of PPIs in causing VAP since the group treated with PPIs included patients with higher levels of seriousness. Those treated with PPIs, therefore, though more serious, had the same incidence of pneumonia compared to patients treated with H_2-receptor antagonists.

Another study published a few years earlier by Levy [35] yielded similar results: the incidence of pneumonia was the same in patients treated with an H_2-receptor antagonist (ranitidine) and a PPI (omeprazole). Even comparing a simple gastric mucosa protector such as sucralfate with antisecretory agents, Yildizdas [36] found the same incidence of VAP in paediatric intensive care.

Even the study published by Cook in 1998 [37] which compared an antisecretory agent (ranitidine) with the usual gastric mucosa protector (sucralfate) in patients receiving mechanical ventilation, there was no difference in the incidence of infections in the two treated groups. In this study, however, the reference antisecretory agent was ranitidine, a H_2-receptor antagonist, which, as we have stated, does not enable increases in gastric pH like PPIs and, unlike these, does not seem to have as many negative effects that affect the immune system.

From this and other data in the literature it can be inferred that the incidence of VAP in critical patients is not clearly influenced by antisecretory treatment with H_2-receptor antagonists and PPIs, which instead is incontrovertible in studies that address nosocomial pneumonia outside intensive care.

How is such a difference possible? It must not be forgotten that this depends on the relatively small number of specimens in studies in ICUs compared to those in hospitalised patients in general. It is sufficient to remember that one study with a higher number of cases in intensive care, led by Cook, was conducted in 2,100 patients whilst a study recently published in *JAMA* by Shoshane included 63,878 patients in non-specialist wards.

Another possible explanation is that ICU patients, due to the seriousness of their conditions, have so many risk factors for pneumonia, which are often simultaneous and interdependent, that it is difficult to provide individual statistics on independent factors such as the inhibition of gastric secretion. If we consider a patient with ample non-ventilated pulmonary regions, as well as ventilated and poorly perfused areas, receiving enteral nutrition with a gastric catheter, mechanical ventilation with orotracheal intubation with frequent tracheal and bronchial suction, with an immune system that is often depressed and multiple organ failure, we realise that identifying an antisecretory strategy as an independent factor in causing pneumonia is anything but easy, especially if, as we have said, the analyses are done on fewer specimens.

We therefore think that, even if studies in critical patients do not provide certain data on the direct relationship between VAP and gastric pH, it would indicate greater responsibility for PPIs versus H$_2$-receptor antagonists in causing VAP, and it would be wise to consider the fundamental work by Shoshane on nosocomial pneumonia that states that PPIs are essential contributors to the occurrence of cases even if this study was not conducted in ICUs.

We are convinced that a review of the use of antisecretory agents in ICUs is indispensible and that, as is happening in non-specialised wards, it is necessary to be more selective when choosing treatment. In this respect the guidelines on the prophylaxis of stress ulcers published in 1999 [38] are still convincing as they recommend prophylaxis in patients with coagulation disorders in those who require mechanical ventilation for more than 48 hours, in those who have had peptic ulcers and/or gastric bleeding in the year before admission.

The same guidelines also recommend the prophylaxis of patients with at least two of the following risk factors: sepsis, more than one week in intensive care, bloody stools for six days or more or hydrocortisone doses higher than 250 mg per day (or equivalent for other corticosteroids). In other patients prophylaxis of stress ulcers is not indicated.

9.4   Conclusion

We have attempted to address in a single chapter the decontamination of the digestive tract and prophylaxis of stress ulcers since the arguments are still under discussion, but a certain agreement has been achieved over the years.

These two therapeutic strategies have different goals: the prevention of VAP for the first and the prevention of stress ulcers for the second. It is not rare that they are activated at the same time.

It is not conceptually wrong and it is even advisable if these strategies are implemented in the correct conditions in suitable patients.

The negative effects that may accompany these treatments must, however, be taken into account: for digestive tract decontamination, above all, the possible selection of multi-resistant microorganisms (which is, however, not documented in studies on the subject) if SDD is used and for the prophylaxis of stress ulcers the possible increase in the incidence of pneumonia, especially when using PPIs.

It appears from more recent literature that digestive tract decontamination can be restricted to the oropharyngeal cavity, without applying a multiple-antibiotic paste but simply by using chlorhexidine.

In terms of the prophylaxis of stress ulcers, it seems to be confirmed, after the important work by Shoshane in the *JAMA* that, in reality, a discrete influence on the incidence of pneumonia can be expected with PPIs, but H$_2$-receptor antagonists play a more minor role, which would be preferable at least when used in non-specialist wards.

Extrapolating this concept to patients in intensive care, as we have said, is not certain but at the moment appears to be a subject of agreement.

Bibliography

1. Guidelines (2005) For the management of adults with hospital-acquired, ventilator associated, and healthcare associated pneumonia. Am J Rest Crit Care Med 171:388-416
2. De Jounge E, Schultz M, Spanjaard l et al (2003) Effect of selective decontamination of the digestive tract on mortality and acquisition of resistant bacteria in intensive care: a randomized, controlled trial. Lancet 362:1011-1016
3. D'Amico R. Pilteri S, Leonetti C et al (1993) Effectiveness of antibiotic prophylaxis in critically ill adult patients: systemic review of randomized controlled trials. BMJ 316:1275-1285
4. Pugin J, Anckenthaler R, Lew DP, Sutter PM (1991) Oropharyngeal decontamination decreases incidence of ventilator-associated pneumonia: a randomized, placebo controlled, double-blind clinical trial. JAMA 265:2704-2710
5. Bergmans DC, Bouten MJ, Gaillard CA et al (2001) Prevention of ventilator associated pneumonia by oral decontamination: a prospective, randomized, double-blind, placebo-controlled study. Am J Resp Crit Care Med 164:382-388
6. Vincent JL (2003) Nosocomial infections in adult intensive care units. Lancet 361:2068-2077
7. Stoutenbeck Cl, Van Saene HKF, Miranda DR et al (1984) The effect of selective decontamination of the digestive tract on colonization and infection rate in multiple trauma patients. Intensive Care Med 10:185-192
8. De La Col MA, Cardà E, Garcia Hierni P et al (2005) Survival benefit in critically ill burned patients receiving selective decontamination of the digestive tract: a randomized, placebo-controlled, double-blind trial. Am Surg 241:424-430
9. Nathans AB, Marshall JC (1999) Selective decontamination of the digestive tract in surgical patients: a systematic review of the evidence. Arch Surg134:170-176
10. Bouten MJM, Gaillard CA, Van Tiel SH et al (1994) The stomach is not a source for colonization of the upper respiratory tract and pneumonia in ICU patients. Chest 105:878-884
11. Garrouste-Orgeas M, Chevret S, Arlet G et al (1997) Oropharyngeal or gastric colonization and nosocomial pneumonia in adult intensive care unit patients: a prospective study based on genomic DNA analysis. Am J Resp Critical Care Med 156:1647-1655.
12. Chan EY, Ruest A, Meade MO et al (2007) Oral decontamination for prevention of pneumonia in mechanically ventilated adults: systematic review and meta-analysis.BMJ 334:889-900
13. Bouten MJ, Kallef MH, Hall JB et al (2004) Risk factors for ventilator-associated pneumonia: from an epidemiology to patient management. Clin Infect Dis 38:1141-1149
14. Guidelines for the management of adults with hospital-acquired, ventilator-associated, and healthcare-associated pneumonia (2005) Am J Resp Crit Care Med 171:388-416
15. De Smet A, Kluytmans J, Cooper RS et al (2009) Decontamination of the digestive tract and oropharynx in ICU patients. N Engl J Med 360:20-31
16. Verwaest C, Verhaegen J, Ferdinande P et al (1997) Randomized controlled trial of selective digestive decontamination in 600 mechanically ventilated patients in multidisciplinary intensive care. Crit Care Med 25:63-71
17. Lingnan W, Berger J, Jaworsky F et al (1998) Changing bacterial ecology during five-year period of selective intestinal decontamination. J Hosp Infect 1998, 39:195-206
18. Hammond JJ, Potgieter PD, Saunders PL et al (1992) Double blind study of selective decontamination of the digestive tract in intensive care. Lancet 340:5-9
19. Koeman M, Van Der Ven AJAM, Hak E et al (2006) Oral decontamination with Chlorhexidine reduces the incidence of ventilator-associated pneumonia. Am J Resp Crit Care Med 173:1348-55
20. Sierra R, Benitez E, Leon C, Rello J (2005) Prevention and diagnosis of ventilator associated pneumonia. Chest 128:1667-1673
21. Heininger A, Meyer E, Schwab F et al (2006) Effects of long-term routine use of SDD on antimicrobial resistance. Intensive Care Med 32:1569-1576
22. Gullotta R, Ferraris L, Cortellezzi C. et al (1997) Are we correctly using the inhibitors of acid

gastric secretion and cytoprotective drugs? Results of a multicentre study. Ital J Gastroent Hepatol 28:325-329

23. Heidelbangh JJ, Inadoerni JM (2006) Magnitude and economic impact of inappropriate use of stress ulcer prophylaxis in non ICU hospitalized patients. Am J Gastroent 101:2200-2205

24. Shoshane JH, Howell MA, Long H et al (2009) Acid suppressive medication use and the risk for Hospital-acquired Pneumonia. JAMA 301:2120-2128

25. Aybay C, Imir T, Okur H (1995) The effect of omeprazole on human Natural Killer cell activity. Gen Pharmacol 26:1413-1418

26. Zedwitz-Liebenstein K, Wenisch C, Patruta S et al (2002) Omeprazole treatment diminish intra and extracellular neutrophil reactive oxygen production and bactericidal activity. Crit. Care Med 300:1118-1122

27. Wandall JH (1992) Effects of omeprazole on neutrophil chemotaxis, super oxide production, degranulation and translocation of cytochrome b 245. Gut 33:617-621

28. Simms HH, Amico RD (1994) Polymorphonuclear leucocyte dysregulation during the systemic inflammatory response syndrome. Blood 83:1398-1407

29. Alexievicz JM, Kurnar D, Smogorrewski M et al (1995) Polymorphonuclear leukocytes in non insulin-dependent diabetes mellitus: abnormalities in metabolism and function. Ann Int Med 123:919-924

30. Wenisch C, Graninger W (1995) Are soluble factors relevant for polymorphonuclear leukocyte dysregulation in septicemia? Clin Diagn Lab Immunol 2:241-245

31. Alexiewicz JM, Smolorrewski M, Fadda GZ et al (1991) Impaired phagocytosis in dialysis patients: studies on mechanisms. Am J Nephrol 11:102-111

32. Mikawa K, Akamatsu H, Nishina K et al (1999) The effect of cimetidine, ranitidine and famotidine on human neutrophil function. Anesth Analg 89:218-224

33. Cook D, Heyland D, Griffith L et al (1999) Risk factors for clinically important upper gastrointestinal bleeding in patients requiring mechanical ventilation. Crit Care Med. 27:2812-2817

34. Mallow S, Rebuck JA, Osler T et al (2004) Do PPI increase the incidence of nosocomial pneumonia and related infections complications when compared with anti H2 receptor antagonists in critically ill patients? Curr Surg 61:452-458

35. Levy MJ, Seelig CB, Robinson NJ et al (1997) Comparison of omeprazole and ranitidine for stress ulcer prophylaxis. Dig Dis Sci 42:1255-1259

36. Yildizdas D, Yapicioglou H, Ylmar HL (2002) Occurrence of VAP in mechanically ventilated pediatric intensive care patients during stress ulcer prophylaxis with sucralfate, ranitidine and omeprazole. J Crit Care 17:240-245

37. Cook D, Guyalt G, Marshall J et al (1998) A comparison of sucralfate and ranitidine for the prevention of upper gastrointestinal bleeding in patients requiring mechanical ventilation. N Eng J Med 338:791-797

38. ASHP Therapeutic guidelines on stress ulcer prophylaxis (1999) Am J Health Syst Pharm 56:347-379

Renal, Cardiac and Pulmonary Involvement in Patients with Supraventricular Tachycardia: a Typical Holistic Vision by an Intensive Care Physician

10

Biagio Allaria

10.1 Introduction

Cases of supraventricular tachycardia are always regarded by anaesthetists as benign forms of arrhythmia that are certainly less dangerous than ventricular arrhythmias. The latter are in fact initially more life-threatening but, but supraventricular tachycardia is not to be completely underestimated since due to its higher incidence rate and often the loss of the body's atrioventricular activation sequence ventricular filling is incomplete, leading to a fall in cardiac output and blood pressure. The resulting haemodynamic imbalance can be dangerous in various regions such as the kidneys, lungs and even the heart from which it originates.

Naturally these imbalances are all the more dangerous the longer they last, and prompt diagnosis and appropriate treatment of arrhythmias are therefore essential.

One organ that is particularly sensitive to the fall in cardiac output associated with these arrhythmias is the kidney, which uses 20% of cardiac output, and in terms of flow for every 100 g of tissue has a flow four times that of the liver and eight times that of the coronary muscle.

Therefore, the kidneys are particularly affected by the fall in cardiac output and blood pressure, even though compensatory mechanisms exist that tend to maintain glomerular filtration and renal plasma flow. The immediate drop in flow caused by tachycardia results in the release of angiotensin that causes vasoconstriction in either the afferent or efferent arterioles, but since the efferent arteriole has a smaller diameter, the increase in efferent arteriole resistance

B. Allaria (✉)
Past Director of Critical Care Department
Istituto Nazionale per lo Studio e la Cura dei Tumori - National Cancer Institute, Milan, Italy
e-mail: biagio.allaria@tiscali.it

caused by angiotensin is three times what it is in the afferent arteriole. This leads to a positive hydraulic effect in the glomerulus and more filtrate. Since, however, extraglomerular renal flow is assured by continuation towards the efferent arteriole tubules, the sharp rise in resistance would lead to a considerable fall in flow if angiotensin II did not stimulate the production of vasodilator prostaglandins that work to maintain flow.

Therefore, if the decrease in pressure and cardiac output caused by tachycardia is not particularly serious and is a short-term effect, the compensatory mechanisms enable acceptable levels of glomerular filtrate and renal flow to be maintained.

But if a patient were treated with an anti-prostaglandin agent (such as an NSAID) and with ACE inhibitors that inhibit angiotensin II production, or an angiotensin-receptor blocker such as a sartan, what would happen? [1] Renal function would certainly be at risk. This example has been cited to help recall that, as well as haemodynamic imbalance caused by arrhythmias, there may be a multiplicity of factors promote dysfunction at a distance.

Similar problems can be confirmed in the coronary muscle, especially with left ventricular load.

It should be remembered that the heart consumes more oxygen in baseline conditions. Studies on closed hearts with maintained coronary circulation have shown that myocardial consumption of baseline oxygen (MVO_2) is 2 mL/100 g/min, which is considerably higher than the skeletal muscle at rest. The MVO_2 of a beating heart is approximately 9 mL/100 g/min at rest and rises substantially with an increase in heart rate.

It is true that heart rate is only one of the determining factors for MVO_2 and that the most important is endoventricular pressure, followed by endoventricular pressure overload. The biggest cause of MVO_2 is therefore pressure overload (for example, aortic stenosis) followed by volume overload (for example, aortic insufficiency) and heart rate. However, when the heart rate is rapid, as with tachycardia, the contribution of heart rate to the increase in MVO_2 can be a relevant factor, especially if the patient is awake and has psychomotor agitation, which often accompanies arrhythmias.

Since left ventricular coronary supply occurs during diastole, which is normally much longer than systole, any reduction in diastole time leads to a fall in coronary flow when a rise in oxygen consumption requires this to increase. This creates a risk of myocardial ischaemia, which is always adjusted when tachycardia occurs.

Coronary circulation too, has a capacity for adjustment and if the coronary endothelium functions regularly, it releases vasodilator substances such as nitric oxide, which enable an acceptable flow even with tachycardia and low diastolic aortic pressure.

But we should be particularly attentive when tachycardia develops in a patient with critical coronary stenosis. In such cases, the poststenotic area is already vasodilated to the maximum in order to enable a sufficient trans-stenotic pressure gradient which maintains flow in basic conditions.

Yet when tachycardia increases myocardial oxygen consumption, downstream from stenosis the compensatory vasodilatation mechanism cannot be activated and flow in this area depends closely on aortic diastolic pressure (which is not the biggest factor for flow in normal conditions) and thus, as mentioned many times, these arrhythmias are often mostly accompanied by hypertension and myocardial ischaemia.

The situation is even more dangerous if the patient has aortic stenosis, which is usually accompanied by diastolic aortic hypotension and an increase in myocardial oxygen consumption and pressure overload. In such cases there is a risk of myocardial ischaemia.

The problem worsens if the patient has endothelial dysfunction, which causes insufficient release of nitric oxide (NO). Endothelial dysfunction is anything but rare since if accompanies very common situations such as tobacco use, diabetes, dyslipidaemia and known coronary disease. In these cases the lack of NO enables endotheline 1, one of the most potent coronary constrictors, which is produced by endothelial cells, to predominate and cause ischaemia. It should be noted that emotional stress which, as we have said, often accompanies these arrhythmias in patients who are awake, is, via the release of catecholamine, an inducer of endotheline release.

It is clear that the more one knows about this, the clearer it is that tachycardia can cause considerable myocardial ischaemia, especially in patients with known coronary stenosis and with confirmed or suspected endothelial dysfunction.

If myocardial ischaemia develops (with a consequent reduction in ventricular compliance), the left atrium normally increases its contraction to maintain ventricular filling and acceptable left ventricular performance [2], but if supraventricular tachycardia is a form of atrial fibrillation, in which the atrial contribution to ventricular filling is lost, the situation becomes dramatic with a subsequent fall in cardiac output and shock.

It is also useful to remember that if myocardial ischaemia is related to stenosis of the anterior descending artery, the atrium will increase its contraction effort to fill the ventricle, but if ischaemia is dependent on proximal stenosis of the circumflex artery, the branches leading from this to the left atrium experience an inevitable fall in flow that also involves atrial ischaemia with the result that the atrium cannot handle the increase in contraction, which would be valuable for maintaining ventricular filling [3].

Another situation in which the loss of atrial supply for cardiac filling is particularly affected is hypertension. The atrial supply for filling becomes very important in cases of diastolic dysfunction of the left ventricle, which is a characteristic of such patients.

It is widely known that the atrium has three functions: it is a reservoir for blood from the pulmonary vein, it passively transfers the blood into the ventricle, and thirdly it "squeezes" the blood into the ventricle with its contractile action. In a hypertensive patient, as well as a reduction in the second function (passive conduction) which is a negative aspect, the other two functions (reservoir and contraction) fortunately increase, ensuring satisfactory filling with no repercussions for pulmonary circulatory pressure (which is the advantage of the increase in the reservoir, which includes a chamber for compensating pressure between the ventricle and pulmonary veins [4].

In hypertensive patients, therefore, the left atrium is larger and the musculature is more hypertrophic, which enables the atrium itself to benefit fully from Starling's law in the contraction phase.

Atrial dilatation in patients with hypertension is a factor that promotes atrial fibrillation (AF) and when this is proven it leads to further dilatation. It triggers a mechanism that leads to frequent episodes of AF. In these patients, therefore, as well as the urgency of normal reconversion of the heart rate to restore valuable atrial supply for ventricular filling, it is necessary to begin basic treatment to reduce diastolic dysfunction: primarily with ACE inhibitors and/or thiazides.

Haemodynamic changes to supraventricular tachycardia, especially in cases characterised by loss of atrial supply for ventricular filling, such as AF and paroxysmal junctional tachycardia, are also felt in the respiratory system via two differing mechanisms. The first involves the previously described difficulty in draining the pulmonary veins in the atrium with resulting pressure in the pulmonary capillary circulation. The increase in hydrostatic pressure in the atrium promotes the transfer of water from the circulation to the interstitium and in particularly serious conditions to the alveoli. Therefore in such cases there is a predisposition to pulmonary oedema which is considerably enhanced if changes also occur to the permeability of the alveolar-capillary barrier (as in patients with sepsis and ARDS) and/or if excessive fluid administration occurs in such situations.

It is known that there is normally a transfer of water from pulmonary capillaries to the interstitium during systole (when capillary hydrostatic pressure is at its highest) and that this water is reabsorbed during diastole, when hydrostatic pressure is lower. Since diastole is longer than systole, the pulmonary interstitium and alveoli are normally dry. It makes sense that this occurs during tachycardia: diastole is shortened considerably while systole varies slightly: this creates a tendency for imbibition of the lungs [5].

The second mechanism that leads to worsening of respiratory exchange is related to the increase in dead space (Vd/Vt). The fall in supply caused by tachycardia reduces pulmonary perfusion by creating a well ventilated but poorly perfused area. This increase in the ventilation/perfusion (V/Q) ratio, and therefore this increase in Vd/Vt, along with the pulmonary oedema previously mentioned, are etiopathogenetic oxygen desaturation factors that often accompany supraventricular tachycardia.

All of this aims to attract our attention to some of the most important changes that may occur with supraventricular tachycardia, especially if it is not promptly recognised or treated.

10.2   Diagnosis

We shall now discuss the most common forms of supraventricular tachycardia in terms of how they are diagnosed and treated.

Diagnosis is essentially by means of an electrocardiogram and, in most cases differential diagnosis between supraventricular and ventricular arrhythmias is based on whether the QRS complex is 'narrow' or 'prolonged'. This difference is due to the fact that in ventricular arrhythmias activation is achieved via different means, causing a prolonged and deformed QRS complex.

Exceptions do exist, however. For example, in a patient with pre-existing bundle branch block, the QRS complex is already prolonged and deformed and therefore, in the event of supraventricular tachycardia the electrocardiographic image is that of ventricular tachycardia. In this case the availability of a pre-existing image showing the presence of bundle branch block with a complete QRS image similar to that of developing tachycardia enables a correct diagnosis to be made easily.

There are also more complex situations in which, even without pre-existing bundle branch block, supraventricular tachycardia occurs with a prolonged QRS complex, imitating ventricular tachycardia. This is so-called supraventricular tachycardia with aberrant ventricular conduction, but in uncertain cases the diagnosis is not within the anaesthetist's competence and it is fully recommended that a cardiologist be consulted.

The other basic point for electrocardiographic diagnosis is the presence or absence of the P wave. It must be remembered that often it is not possible to identify the P wave in monitoring leads and that therefore it is advisable to perform an ECG using twelve leads. The leads in which the P wave are most clearly visible are D2, D3, aVF and V1. Identification of the P wave is important for the differential diagnosis between uniform atrial tachycardia (UAT) and multiform atrial tachycardia (MAT) (Fig. 10.1). Both are relatively more common in children and rarer in adults. a heart rate of 100-250 beats per minute is reached. The former has completely uniform P waves, the latter has P waves with varying morphology. MAT is caused by changes to ectopic foci in the atrium, and more commonly occurs in critical or elderly patients and those with pulmonary disease [6]. In the case of reentrant arrhythmia, for example with UAT, arrhythmia begins and ends abruptly.

In paroxysmal supraventricular tachycardia caused by a re-entry mechanism in the atrioventricular node, episodes begin and end suddenly and the morphology of the P wave that initiates the crisis is generally different from that of successive P waves. This form of tachycardia has a rate of 120 to 300 beats per minute and affects children and young adults with no cardiac disease.

Finally it is important to check whether tachycardia is regular or irregular. This enables differentiation between forms of paroxysmal supraventricular tachycardia such as nodal reentrant tachycardia, atrial tachycardia, accessory

ATRIAL FIBRILLATION (AF)
ATRIAL FLUTTER (AFL)

In AF the R-R intervals on the ECG change continually

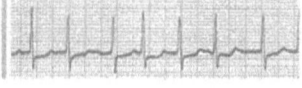
P waves are entirely irregular and reduced to slight undulations (fine fibrillation) or larger undulations (coarse fibrillation). Ventricular frequency ranges from 100 to 200.

In AFL the R-R intervals vary the most

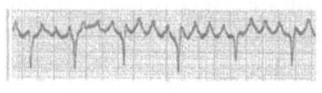
P waves are clearly visible in V₁ and often look like the teeth of a saw. Ventricular frequency ranges from 100 to 200. The most common frequency is ~140.

Fig. 10.1 Irregular narrow QRS tachycardia

tachycardia and junctional tachycardia, which are primarily 'regular' (i.e. with minimal R-R variation), from those such as AF and atrial flutter (in which the difference between one R-R interval and another can exceed 20 ms), which have a narrow but 'irregular' QRS complex.

The concept of distinguishing between 'regular' from 'irregular' tachycardia is fundamental when considering treatment.

10.3   Treatment

In regular tachycardia the very first goal is to interrupt arrhythmia (using ordinary vagal manoeuvres such as compression of the carotid artery and/or administration of adenosine) (Fig. 10.2).

The recommended adenosine dose is 6 mg as a rapid bolus administration in an antecubital vein followed by 20 mL of normal saline solution also as a rapid bolus administration, immediately upon raising the arm. The aim of this is for the drug to reach the heart as quickly as possible, considering how fast it is metabolised. If this fails a second bolus may be tried with a double dose (12 mg) after two minutes and possibly another bolus administration of 12 mg two minutes after that [7]. A similar success rate can be obtained with amiodarone, which we shall discuss below.

In irregular tachycardias (such as AF and AFL) (Fig. 10.1) the most urgent objective is to reduce heart rate by enabling more suitable ventricular filling (i.e. with small bolus amounts of beta-blockers, such as 1 mg of metoprolol per minute for 5 minutes until a maximum of 15 mg is reached, or 0.25 mg/kg of diltiazem followed if necessary by a second bolus of 0.35 mg/kg). It is believed

a) with vagal manoeuvres

b) with drugs:

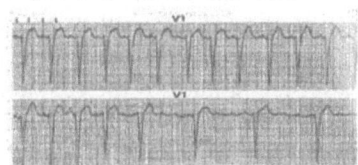

> ➤ Adenosine 6 mg as a rapid bolus administration – in an antecubital vein followed by 20 ml of a normal saline solution immediately upon raising the arm.
> If unsuccessful, after 2 minutes: double dose (12 mg)
> ➤ Amiodarone 150 mg (1 vial) over 10 minutes
> then 1 mg/ml for 6 hours

Fig. 10.2 Regular narrow QRS tachycardia

that if AF or AFL occur in patients with known WPW syndrome, diltiazem or another calcium channel blocker such as verapamil is absolutely not suggested.

With a reduction in heart rate and relative haemodynamic reorganisation the recovery of the atrial component in cardiac filling that re-establishes sinus rhythm does not need to be abandoned. This can be achieved with various drugs. In particular we should advise that, among other thing, they can also be used as first-line treatment to reduce heart rate: amiodarone and ibutilide (which can also be used in patients with WPW syndrome).

Amiodarone is a complex drug that acts on Na, K and Ca channels as well as having a blocking action on alpha and beta-adrenergic cells. It is preferred to other anti-arrhythmics in patients with manifest cardiac insufficiency. The recommended dose is 150 mg as an infusion lasting ten minutes, followed by 1 mg/min for six hours and then 0.5 mg/min for a further 18 hours as maintenance treatment. Doses can be increased if there is resistance to 2.2 g over a 24-hour period (fourteen vials of the commercially available product). The effect on heart rate in patients with AF is rapid, but the restoration of sinus rhythm is slower and generally occurs after four or six hours [7].

Ibutilide is an anti-arrhythmic agent with a short duration of action which prolongs the action potential and refractory period of the cardiac tissue. It can be used, as we have said, to reduce heart rate in patients with AF and to re-establish sinus rhythm even in those with WPW syndrome (in whom, however, the treatment of choice would be cardioversion). It is possibly the most effective anti-arrhythmic for the restoration of sinus rhythm in patients with recent AF, but it must be remembered that cases of ventricular arrhythmia are common (ventricular tachycardia, torsades de pointes) with this drug and that prior to administration it is important to correct possible hypokalaemia and hypomagnesaemia. When using ibutilide, therefore, continuous monitoring is vital during administration and for at least four to six hours afterwards. The drug is contraindicated if the QT interval exceeds 0.44 seconds. For an adult weighing more than 60 kg the dose is 1 mg intravenously over ten minutes, which can be repeated after ten minutes if the first dose is unsuccessful. In patients weighing less than 60 kg, the recommended dose is 0.01 mg/kg [7].

In Italy verapamil is still commonly used to interrupt regular paroxysmal supraventricular tachycardia that is reentrant or automatic (junctional, atrial) or to reduce heart rate in patients with AF and AFL. It should, however, be pointed out that this drug is contraindicated in patients with WPW syndrome and a history of cardiac insufficiency. The initial verapamil dose is between 2.5 mg and 5 mg over two minutes (½ to 1 vial of the commercially available product), repeated if necessary at a dose of 5 mg to 10 mg (½ to 1 vial) every thirty minutes until a maximum dose of 20 mg (4 vials) is achieved.

Propafenone is just as commonly used, restoring sinus rhythm in patients with AF in a similar way to amiodarone (80%), but with the advantage of achieving the objective in a shorter time. The recommended dose is 2 mg/kg as a bolus administration, followed by 20 mg/kg over a 24-hour period. Yet amiodarone has a lower effect on heart rate, which, as we have seen, is the most important feature in the first moments of treatment [11].

However, it seems to have been confirmed that in anaesthesiology and interventional surgery, for all tachycardias, whether regular or irregular, amiodarone can be considered a drug of choice. In fact, it is least depressant in cases of cardiac insufficiency, rapidly reduces heart rate within a few minutes of treatment, has a good success rate in restoring sinus rhythm, is not contraindicated in patients with WPW syndrome, and in cases of tachycardia with a prolonged QRS complex of uncertain etiology it is effective in both supraventricular and ventricular arrhythmias.

Finally, it is worth mentioning electric cardioversion of supraventricular tachycardia. The main indication for cardioversion is haemodynamic instability. In patients with severe instability this procedure is indispensible because it enables sinus rhythm to be restored quickly without administering cardiodepressant drugs, which is what all anti-arrhythmic agents are.

It should, however be remembered that regular paroxysmal automatic tachycardias (junctional and multifocal atrial tachycardia) are mostly not susceptible to electric cardioversion, whereas regular paroxysmal reentrant supraventricular tachycardias are.

Therefore, before applying electrical cardioversion in patients with regular paroxysmal supraventricular tachycardia, anaesthetists should consult a cardiologist and should use therapeutic approaches that are not dangerous, such as vagal stimulation and administration of adenosine.

In the case of irregular tachycardias (AF and AFL) with marked haemodynamic instability there is no doubt: electric cardioversion should be used and synchronised with the QRS complex to avoid a decrease in discharge in "vulnerable periods" of the cardiac cycle, where shock may cause ventricular fibrillation, especially with a low-energy discharge that is used in supraventricular tachycardia [8].

The recommended discharge energy varies in the case of monophasic and biphasic defibrillation: for the former it is 100-200 J, for the latter it is lower (100-120 J). Successive discharges with higher energy are possible if the first is ineffective.

10.4 Conclusions

Supraventricular tachycardia is a major problem for anaesthetists and providers of resuscitation, especially following surgery.

A relatively recent study in 4,181 patients undergoing non-cardiac elective surgery revealed supraventricular tachycardia in 317 patients [9]. The factors that promoted arrhythmias were: type of surgery (especially pulmonary and aortic surgery), history of the same type of arrhythmia, valve disease, or a concomitant disease unrelated to surgery (such as pneumonia, gastrointestinal haemorrhage and bacteraemia). The presence of arrhythmia increased LOS by 33%.

It is possible to predict the onset of these arrhythmias, especially with atrial fibrillation, which is the most common form. Leung et al. [10] used transoesophageal echocardiography to study 300 patients and demonstrated a relationship between the incidence of postoperative atrial fibrillation and an increase in the size of the left atrium and left auricle, as well as a reduction in the atrial ejection fraction and diastolic dysfunction of the left ventricle. These are common changes in elderly patients, especially those with hypertension, which we described at the beginning of this review. A preliminary echocardiographic study of atrial function and left ventricular diastolic function would be useful to enable the selection of patients who are more prone to developing this type of arrhythmia after surgery, and also to enable implementation of all measures to avoid co-factors that may promote the onset (hypokalaemia, hypomagnesaemia, fluid overloading, hypoxaemia especially after surgery, adrenergic stimuli such as postoperative pain that is not treated properly, and abnormal myocardial consumption of oxygen as with postoperative shivering, etc.).

The haemodynamic repercussions of arrhythmia in the kidneys, heart and lungs fully justify the 33% increase in LOS to which we referred.

Renal, coronary and pulmonary repercussions of arrhythmias, which are often underestimated in anaesthesia, deserve special attention in terms of prognosis, diagnosis and treatment.

Bibliography

1. Rose BD, Post TW (2001) Clinical physiology of acid base and electrolyte disorders, McGraw-Hill, New York
2. Sigwart H, Garby MM, Gay J, Kappenberger L (1990) Left atrial function in acute transient left ventricular ischemia produced during percutaneous transluminal coronary angioplasty of the left anterior descending coronary artery. Am J Cardiol 65:282-286

3.   Keren A, De Anda A, Korned M et al (1995) Pitfalls in creation of left atrial pressure-area relationships with automated border detection. J Am Soc Echocardiog 8:169-178
4.   Stefanadis C, Toutouras DP (2001) A clinical appraisal of left atrial function. European Heart Journal, 22:22-36
5.   Lee G de J, (1994) Studies of the lung-microcirculation. In: Wagner WW, Weir EK, The pulmonary circulation and gas exchange, pp. 189-219. Futura, New York
6.   Atlee JL (1997) Perioperative cardiac dysrhythmias: diagnosis and management. Anesthesiology 86:1394-1424
7.   ACC/AHA/ESC (2003) Guidelines for the management of patients with supraventricular tachycardias. Circulation 108:1871-1909
8.   Town B (1967) Electrical reversion of cardiac arrhythmias. Br Heart J 29:469-489
9.   Shammash JB, Ghali WA (2003) Preoperative assessment and perioperative management of the patient with nonischemic heart disease. Med Clin N Am 87:137-152
10. Leung JM, Bellows WH, Schiller NB (2004) Impairment of left atrial function predicts postoperative atrial fibrillation after coronary artery bypass graft surgery. Europ Heart J 25:1836-1844
11. Plinter A et al (2001) Intravenous antiarrhythmic agents. Current Opinion in Critical Care 16:17-22

VAP (Ventilator-Associated Pneumonia)

Davide Chiumello and Tommaso Fossali

11.1 Definition and Pathogenesis

Pneumonia is the presence of infectious flogistic infiltrate in the pulmonary parenchyma. The type of pneumonia observed in intensive care patients is mainly caused by inhalation of micro-organisms found in oral, rhinonopharyngeal or gastro-intestinal flora. The micro-organisms reach distal airways when the defences of the upper respiratory tract become altered (coma, surgery) or when endotracheal tube or treacheostomy cannula are in place. The lower respiratory tract is in fact maintained in a sterile state by a variety of defence mechanisms: glottis as a natural anatomical barrier, cough reflex, bronchial secretion combined with ciliary movement, cell-mediated and humoral immunity and phagocytic activity of alveolar macrophages and neutrophils. The onset of pneumonia starts when micro-organisms succeed in clearing these barriers and in reaching the pulmonary parenchyma due to a flaw in the host's defences, to their own particular virulence or to an overwhelming infiltration [1, 2].

The actual "VAP" definition has lately been the subject of doubt since the most directly implicated factor is not mechanical ventilation per se but the procedure of intubation instead and the presence of tube and cannula in the airways. It would seem therefore more appropriate to re-name it "intubation-associated pneumonia" in case of early onset and "tube-associated pneumonia" in case of delayed onset [3, 4].

Onset timing is of the utmost importance. VAP is usually classified as follows:

D. Chiumello (✉)
Department of Anesthesiology, Resuscitation and Pain Medicine
Fondazione IRCCS Ca' Granda Ospedale Maggiore Policlinico, Milan, Italy
chiumello@libero.it

Biagio Allaria (ed.), *Practical Issues in Anesthesia and Intensive Care*
© Springer-Verlag Italia 2012

- early onset when it develops 4-5 days from intubation;
- late onset when it develops after 5 days.

This distinction is significant when considering aetiologic agents, seriousness and prognosis. The exact interval for establishing early or late onset varies, according to published literature, between 3 and 7 days but the basic concept is that the patient's oropharyngeal bacteria at the time of intubation are most likely the cause of early onset. With each passing day, more virulent and antibiotic-resistant bacteria in the intensive care unit also play a role. It is also important to take into account the admission date in relation to the date of intubation since it is more likely that hospital pathogens colonise a patient a few days after admission [5].

11.2   Epidemiology and Risk Factors

The lack of universally recognized diagnostic criteria is an obstacle to the collection of accurate data and the absence of a gold standard raises controversy with regard to adequacy and relevance of many current studies.

VAP is classified in the nosocomial pneumonia group with a total incidence of approximately 9-10%. Intubated and mechanically ventilated patients have a massively increased risk (10 to 20 times higher) to develop pneumonia compared to non-intubated patients.

VAP incidence in intensive care patients is reported as varying between 8 and 28% [6] and the incidence increases along with each progressive day on mechanical ventilation [7]. Incremental risk of pneumonia related to the progressive number of days on mechanical ventilation varies from study to study since it depends on the characteristics of the population under exam, on concurrent disease and on antibiotics use. Some studies mention a daily 1% risk rise for each day, others report a massive rise during the first 5-7 days with the risk levelling off and remaining constant afterwards [8]. VAP is a common complication of acute respiratory distress syndrome (ARDS) affecting 34 to 70% of these patients; it may lead to sepsis, multiple organ failure and death. The higher incidence can be attributed to the significant changes in pulmonary cells in the course of ARDS, especially immune response. In vitro tests have in fact shown that alveolar macrophages and neutrophils have a low phagocytic ability and reduced activity even after adequate stimulation [9].

Reported mortality is between 24 and 76% and the relative risk is between 1.7 and 4.4 compared to non-VAP patients. Despite statistics underlining how serious VAP pathology is, it has not been clearly proved that VAP is the main cause of death in these patients because it is somewhat difficult to identify a pneumonia patient with total certainty but mainly because many clinical conditions predispose a patient to contracting VAP. It is difficult to establish which, between the severe initial disease and the subsequent pneumonia, has more impact on mortality and we cannot establish that the same patients would survive if they had not developed VAP. Pneumonia certainly affects prognosis to a great extent for some groups of patients, such as post-cardiac-surgery patients, immunocompromised patients, patients who received lung or bone marrow transplant. VAP does not significantly affect prognosis for young patients without any co-morbidity or for cardiac arrest or trauma survivors. Many factors support the fact that the presence of pulmonary infection is an essential component of a poor prognosis for a VAP patient [10].

VAP patient mortality risk factors have been studied by means of multiple linear regression analysis and it has been noted that prognosis is negatively affected by: worsening respiratory failure, progression of underlying condition, shock, inappropriate antibiotic therapy, type of intensive care treatment [11].

Prognosis for aerobic Gram-negative bacteria-induced VAP is significantly worse than for Gram-positive bacterial infection when the latter is antibiotic-sensitive. Mortality rate associated to Pseudomonas aeruginosa is 70-80% according to one study, whereas other studies report 87% mortality with Pseudomonas and Acinetobacter when compared to a rate of 55% for other pathogens. Mortality for MRSA (Methicillin-resistant Staphylococcus aureus) pneumonia is 86% to the rate of 12% for MSSA (Methicillin-sensitive Staphylococcus aureus) with a relative death risk of 20.

11.3 Aetiologic Agents: Microbiology

Aetiologic agents may vary depending on patient's characteristics, on length of hospital and intensive care stay and also on the diagnostic methods employed. The most frequently observed micro-organisms (60%) are Gram-negative bacteria such as Pseudomonas aeruginosa, Escherichia coli, Klebsiella pneumoniae, Acinetobacter baumannii (Table 11.1). There has recently been an increase in Gram-positive bacteria-induced pneumonia (30%) with Staphylococcus aureus as the main agent [12].

Table 11.1 Main aetiological agents and respective incidence

Gram-negative	Pseudomonas aeruginosa	24.4%
	Acinetobacter baumannii	7.9%
	Stenotrophomonas maltophilia	1.7%
	Enterobacter spp	14.1%
	Klebsiella pneumoniae	2.1%
	Escherichia coli	3.3%
	Proteus spp	3.1
	Haemophilus influenzae	9.8%
Gram-positive	Staphylococcus aureus	20.4%
	Streptococcus spp	8.0%
	Streptococcus pneumoniae	4.1%

Between 13 and 40% of patients present a polymicrobial infection. Underlying conditions may be a predisposing factor to contracting an infection by a specific agent. COPD patients have a higher risk of Moraxella catarrhalis, Haemophilus influenzae or Streptococcus pneumoniae while cystic fibrosis increases risk of Pseudomonas; trauma and neurological patients are instead more exposed to Staphylococcus aureus.

Micro-organisms also vary depending on the time of onset. H. influenzae, S. pneumoniae, MSSA or antibiotic-sensitive Enterobacteriaceae are more frequent in early-onset-VAP while late-onset-VAP patients are prey to MRSA and multiresistant Gram-negative bacteria. This difference in distribution is also due to the fact that patients developing late VAP have often been treated with antibiotics whilst admitted and such therapy causes a selection of resistant bacteria to take hold. Prolonged stay in intensive care also promotes colonisation by environmental microbial flora. Any previous antibiotic therapy must be considered when evaluating also early VAP patients since multiresistant bacteria are more likely to be present [13].

Further predisposing factors to pneumonia have been identified within the group of mechanically ventilated patients; the awareness of risk factors makes it possible to identify which patients are more susceptible so that preventive measures can be taken. Table 11.2 shows independent risk factors that were identified by multivariate analysis.

Table 11.2 Independent VAP-inducing risk factors

Patient-related factors	Treatment-related factors
Albumin < 2.2 g/dL	Proton pump inhibitors
Age > 60 years	Sedation and muscle paralysis
ARDS	Transfusion > 4 units
COPD, chronic pulmonary disease	Intracranial pressure monitoring
Coma or altered awareness	Invasive ventilation > 2 days
Trauma or burns	PEEP
Organ failure	Frequent circuit replacement
Seriousness of disease	Re-intubation
High-volume gastric aspiration	Nasogastric tube
Acidity and gastric colonisation	Supine position
Colonisation of upper respiratory airways	Transport outside intensive care unit
Sinusitis	Previous antibiotic therapy

- *Surgery*: Approximately one third of VAP diagnoses concern patients admitted after surgery. Pneumonia is mainly observed in patients with a high perioperative risk marker, i.e. patients with low albumin concentration and high ASA score. Lengthy thoracic and upper abdomen surgical procedures also put older patients (> 65 years) and smokers (> 40 cigarettes/day) at risk.

- *Endotracheal tube and tracheostomy*: The endotracheal tube significantly lowers the airways defences when it creates a by-pass of the glottis; the tube also causes localised inflammation. Micro-leaks around the cuff also allow secretions to pass into the trachea, it is therefore extremely important to carry out frequent checks on filling pressure [14].

  An exam by electronic microscope has revealed that the tube itself is covered and colonised by bacteria which form a true bacterial biofilm covering the entire surface. One hypothesis is that it originates during bronchial aspiration to dislocate bacteria and the bacteria, once on the tube walls, grow unchallenged by the patient's defence mechanisms.

  Re-intubation is a further risk factor possibly due to a higher risk of inhalation in those patients who have been intubated for days, who may be in a state of altered awareness or who have yet to regain complete control and defences of the airways; or the risk could be indirect aspiration of gastric material especially when a nasogastric tube is in place.

  The link between VAP and tracheostomy is the subject of discussion. In theory the tracheostomy cannula, by keeping the vocal chords free, lowers the risk of inhalation of oropharyngeal secretions and prevents microtrauma and oedema of the glottic region. Bacterial biofilm normally settling on the endotracheal tube, which is a real reservoir of micro-organisms, would also be reduced. Tracheotomy finally promotes weaning thus reducing the interval of exposure to VAP. These theoretical suppositions are so far lacking clinical study confirmation. The incidence of VAP with and without tracheostomy has not been compared and there are conflicting results with regard to timing and to surgical versus percutaneous procedures.

- *Antibiotic therapy*: The use of antibiotics in the hospital environment is associated with an increased risk of pneumonia and of selection by resistant micro-organisms. Prophylactic use of antibiotics in intensive care promotes the onset of superinfections by resistant pathogens; this practice fails to fend off hospital infections, it merely delays their onset.

- *Stress ulcer prophylaxis*: Many studies have demonstrated the direct link between gastric alkalinisation and bacterial colonisation and how normal stomach acidity, usually pH < 2, prevents bacterial growth.

- *Nasogastric tube / Enteral feeding*: The presence of a nasogastric tube may increase oropharyngeal colonisation, the pooling of secretions, reflux and aspiration. The early start of enteral feeding is a positive fact for the critical patient but it can also promote gastric colonisation, gastro-oesophageal reflux, aspiration and pneumonia; the patient's supine position with the head lying flat is also a contributing factor.

- *Breathing circuit*: Ventilator parts, especially the connecting tubes, are a possible source of infection due to humidity and condensation being the ideal conditions for bacterial growth. It has been observed that even a frequent circuit replacement routine does not actually prevent VAP.

- *Sinusitis*: Patients suffering from infectious sinusitis are more predisposed to developing VAP. It would appear that orotracheal intubation should be preferred to nasotracheal intubation since the latter could promote the onset of sinusitis.

11.4 Diagnosis

The diagnostic strategy aims to identify patients at high risk of pneumonia so that an adequate antibiotic therapy can be initiated without delay; to delay such therapy would have a negative impact on mortality. The timing and the choice of adequate treatment are the cornerstones on which a favourable outcome rests.

The certainty that a bacterial focus of infection is present in the pulmonary parenchyma can be reached exclusively by histological examination after lung biopsy which, for obvious reasons, is not easily feasible. Diagnosis therefore rests on a combination of three factors: clinical signs of infection, radiological signs of pneumonia, microbiological proof of bacterial colonisation.

The clinical approach follows criteria indicating a high probability of pneumonia and therefore the necessity of initiating empirical antibiotic therapy. The criteria are as follows: presence of newly developed infiltrate on the chest X-ray together with one of the following clinical signs:

- fever (T > 38°C) or hypothermia (T < 36°C);
- leukocytosis or leukopenia;
- considerable and purulent secretions.

Systemic signs of infection are non-specific, they are instead a common finding in any condition where circulating cytokines are released, i.e. in all SIRS cases and, in intensive care, SIRS is very frequent, for instance in trauma and burns patients or in the postoperative period.

With regard to chest X-ray, the presence of infiltrate can be observed also with pulmonary oedema, contusion, atelectasis and it is therefore more useful when negative so that pneumonia can be excluded. The presence of aerial bronchograms is a highly predictive sign though it is non-specific for ARDS patients [15].

Microbiological diagnosis not only confirms the presence of bacteria in the bronchial tree but it can also identify the pathogen and so lead to a targeted therapy. Examination by microscope, or by culture, of bronchial secretions or sputum, the so-called qualitative approach, produces a high percentage of false positive results and it is therefore inconclusive for a pneumonia diagnosis since the upper respiratory tract of many intensive care patients is colonised by pathogens even if there is no underlying infection.

The quantitative approach is the most accurate in reaching a diagnosis and it is based on the fact that the growth of a certain quantity of bacterial colonies in the tracheal aspirate culture is linked to the presence of pulmonary infection. Normal cut-off for bronchial aspirate is 10^6 cfu/mL, for bronchoalveolar lavage (BAL) it is 10^4 cfu/mL and for protected specimen brush (PSB) it is 10^3 cfu/mL. Specimen collection from distal airways by non-bronchoscopic technique is a non-invasive, easier to perform, less costly, low-impact procedure that also has little influence on respiratory exchange and it can also be performed with tracheal tubes of small diameter. Disadvantages are sampling errors due to the blind technique and lack of visual aid while a bronchoscope would be guided to the collection site.

Recent studies demonstrate that bronchoscopic and non-bronchoscopic techniques are equivalent with regard to accuracy in obtaining a specimen from the distal airways, in evaluating outcome and in deciding on antibiotic total use. It is recommended to use the technique dictated by the expertise and resources available at that particular hospital [16].

VAP clinical signs are therefore not very specific but even when diagnosis is not absolutely certain it is reasonable to initiate empirical therapy as soon as possible especially in those cases when the patient's life is at risk, e.g. in the presence of septic compromise or deterioration of gas exchange. This approach results in part of the patients being treated, without any actual need, with antibiotic therapy mandated by false positive results; in order to avoid excessive use of antibiotics it is imperative to re-assess the presence of VAP after 48-72 hours of treatment so that unhelpful and hence harmful administration can be stopped if VAP appears not be likely. Withdrawal of treatment must satisfy three criteria:
1. unlikely clinical diagnosis (X-ray shows no infiltration and just one of the following elements is present: fever, lekocytosis, purulent secretions);
2. the results of tracheobronchial specimens' culture are not significative
3. absence of severe sepsis or septic shock.

11.5 Treatment

VAP treatment remains a multi-faceted challenge and success is by no means assured. Despite VAP being a much studied disease, the ideal treatment is still elusive because there are no universally accepted criteria pointing to a definite diagnosis, because methods vary a great deal and because there is no technique for accurately and precisely monitor the effect of antibiotic therapy on in situ bacterial growth.

11.5.1 Empirical Treatment

It is of the utmost importance to start appropriate antibiotic therapy in order to increase survival. An inappropriate selection of initial antibiotic treatment has in fact demonstrated to be linked to higher mortality and to a risk 5.8 times higher even when treatment is adjusted and modified on the basis of microbiological results. On the other hand antibiotic treatment is not risk-free and can potentially be harmful since it stimulates bacterial selection which in turn promotes colonisation and superinfection by resistant bacteria. This effect can be observed both short and long-term and concerns not only the affected patient but also the entire intensive care and hospital environment. Any therapeutic treatment exerts a particular selective action on local flora so the choice of empirical treatment must also take into account different pathogens and resistance typical of that particular location. The problem of bacterial resistance is becoming more and more widespread and the microbiological trend is evolving towards progressively more resistant and more difficult to treat bacteria; for this reason wide-spectrum empirical treatment may not be sufficient to protect against highly resistant bacteria such as extended-spectrum beta-lactamase-producing (ESBL) Gram-negative bacilli. Microbiological results of previous cultures may assist in selecting empirical treatment despite the fact that bacteria found earlier in the airways is not always the aetiologic agent responsible for the ensuing pneumonia; when colonisation by a multiresistant bacterium is present, however, the risk of an infection caused by that same bacterium is higher [17].

Empiric treatment selection requires a thorough evaluation of the clinical state because the clinical state leads to identification of possible risk factors and of possible presence of various pathogens and their resistance patterns.

The three determining factors are:
1. the patient is either breathing spontaneously or is under ventilation;
2. onset timing (early vs. late onset);
3. risk factors (age, structural lung disease, previous antibiotic therapy, previous tracheal colonisation.)

Empiric treatment guidelines categorise patients on the basis of onset timing (early vs. late) and of risk factors presence or absence (Tables 11.3-11.5).

The results of direct microscopic examination of bronchial secretions are an important evaluation tool during the initial stage and before culture results become available since not only can they confirm VAP diagnosis but they also identify micro-organisms' Gram and morphology thus giving indication as to which specific therapeutic regimen should be initiated.

Table 11.3 Empirical treatment of early-onset VAP

Early-onset pneumonia and no risk factors (one of the following drugs)	
Aminopenicillin + β-latctamase inhibitor	Amoxicillin-clavulanic acid 2.2 g x 3 Ampicillin-sulbactam 3 g x 3
Second-generation Cephalosporin	Cefuroxime 1.5 g x 3
Third-generation Cephalosporin	Cefotaxime 2 g x 3 Ceftriaxone 2 g x 1
"Respiratory" quinolone (not Ciprofloxacin)	Levofloxacin 750 mg x 1 Moxifloxacin 400 mg x 1

Table 11.4 Empirical treatment of late-onset VAP

Late-onset pneumonia (β-lactamin of own choice + quinolone of own choice + anti-MRSA if necessary)	
Piperacillin-tazobactam	4.5 g x 3
Ceftazidime	2 g x 3
Imipenem/Cilastatin	1 g x 3
Meropenem	1 g x 3
+	
Ciprofloxacin	400 mg x 3
Levofloxacin	750 mg x 1
for suspected MRSA	
Vancomycin	1 g x 2
Linezolid	600 mg x 2

Table 11.5 Empirical treatment of both early and late-onset VAP when risk factors are present

Pneumonia with risk factors	
MRSA	Vancomicin 1 g x 2
	Linezolid 600 mg x 2
Peudomonas aeruginosa	anti-*Pseudomonas* combination treatment (see late-onset pneumonia treatment)
Acinetobacter spp	Imipenem-cilastatin 1 g x 3
	Meropenem 1 g x 3
	Ampicillin-sulbactam 3 g x 3
Legionellosis	"Respiratory" quinolone
Mycotic infections	Fluconazole 800 mg x 2
	Caspofungin 70 mg x 1 (loading dose, thereafter 50 mg x 1)
	Voriconazole 4 mg/kg (for suspected *Aspergillus*)

11.5.2 Selection of Drugs

In vitro testing of bacteria and antimicrobial agents interactions is of great assistance in selecting which drugs to administer. Each molecule's characteristics and its ability to act on bacteria at pulmonary level must however be carefully considered.

- *Aminoglycosides*: This group is more active on some Gram-negative strains than some β-lactam antibiotics and has several added advantages: bactericidal properties, concentration-dependence, persistent effects and synergy with β-lactam antibiotics. The disadvantages are low penetration capability into the lung tissue and deactivation due to infected airway low pH all of which hampers any bactericidal activity; for these reasons Aminoglycosides are always used in combination with β-lactam antibiotics.

- *Cephalosporins*: Third and fourth generation cephalosporins may be divided into two groups depending on their efficacy against *Pseudomonas aeruginosa*. Ceftazidime is very effective against *Pseudomonas* but not at all against *Staphylococcus aureus*; on the contrary Ceftriaxone and Cefotaxime have good activity against *Staphylococcus* but poor activity against *Pseudomonas*.

- *Imipenem-meropenem*: Imipenem is an ultra-broad spectrum antibiotic and is active against most Gram-positive bacteria (except for MRSA and enterococci) and against most Gram-negative bacteria including *Pseudomonas* and also most anaerobes. Insurgence of resistance episodes has however been reported and epileptic crisis in the course of treatment has also been mentioned especially in the presence of renal failure. Meropenem has a similar spectrum to Imipenem but it is less active against Gram-positive and more active against Gram-negative bacteria; it also has lower renal and epileptogenic toxicity.

- *Fluoroquinolones*: This group has excellent intracellular concentration capability in most of the tissues including bronchial mucosa, neutrophils and alveolar macrophages possibly resulting in increased efficacy against intermediate sensitivity pathogens.

The efficacy of antibiotic treatment depends not only on the selection of the right molecule but also on its adequate release at the effector site; sub-optimal dosage represents a risk factor for resistance insurgence during treatment and the greatest care must be taken to ensure optimal dosage, method and timing of administration.

Consideration must also be given to pharmacokinetics and dynamics and to the characteristics of time-dependence and concentration-dependence as well as to tissue penetration capability since any therapeutic efficacy is only obtained if antibiotic levels in the infected tissue are equal to at least the pathogen's MIC. Aminoglycosides for instance have a lung tissue penetration capability of 30-40% while ß-lactam antibiotics' index is < 50%; quinolones have a 100% tissue concentration compared to plasma concentration. With regard to Vancomycin, it has been observed that continuous infusion of 20-30 mg/mL is superior to intermittent bolus doses [1, 4].

There are limited data on antimicrobials administration by respiratory route, tracheal instillation or inhalation in combination or not with a systemic therapy. Antimicrobial therapy by inhalation, despite being a promising method, should at present be used only as the alternative therapeutic last resort for VAP cases induced by Gram-negative *Enterobacter* or multiresistant *Pseudomonas aeruginosa*.

11.5.3 Mono Therapy vs. Combination Therapy

Recent studies have shown that monotherapy is not superior to combination therapy in terms of either outcome or onset of resistance. It is currently deemed appropriate for a combination therapy to only be administered in the initial stages i.e. in the first 48 hours as it reduces the risk of inadequate treatment, a notorious cause of excessive mortality. Once the pathogen sensitivity has been established, it is suggested to switch to monotherapy which has shown not to be inferior to combination therapy [18].

11.5.4 De-escalation

As the results of airway secretion cultures or haemocultures become available and confirm individual pathogens' type and corresponding antibiogram, the antibiotic spectrum must be narrowed down and the antibiotic targeted to the pathogen that has been identified; targeted treatment means a lesser use of antibiotics without prejudice to treatment quality. For most patients the treatment should be scaled down to monotherapy from day 3 to day 5 once it is established that the initial therapy had been adequate, that the clinical course is improving and therefore that the patient is responding to treatment and once also established that microbiological data do not point to truly difficult to treat micro-organisms.

11.5.5 Duration of Treatment

VAP antibiotic therapy should last 8 days; a prolonged treatment leads to colonisation by resistant bacteria which in turn may cause relapse or recurrent episodes and added disadvantages are drug toxicity and high cost. Antibiotics represent 20 to 50% of a hospital pharmaceutical expenditure and overuse promotes more resistant bacterial strains which require broader spectrum antibiotics that are usually very costly.

On the other hand a treatment that has not been sufficiently prolonged results in therapeutic failure and relapse, both of which find confirmation in the reappearance of pneumonia clinical signs and in the isolation of the same previous pathogen that, in the meantime, may or may not have acquired resistance. The 8-day duration does not apply to MRSA infection, to immunocompromised patients, to patients whose initial treatment proved inadequate and to patients infected by a difficult to treat micro-organism; caution suggests that the last group of patients be switched to a different antibiotic therapy on the eighth day in view of prolonged treatment [19].

Treatment efficacy monitoring requires, besides clinical signs, serum markers such as procalcitonin and PCR testing; the results provide assistance when deciding to interrupt antibiotic treatment.

11.5.6 Treatment Failure

A failed response to the initial treatment is a worrying occurrence linked to a high incidence of unfavourable outcome which is to be expected in 20-40% of these cases also depending on the seriousness of pneumonia and of any concurrent diseases. Each therapeutic failure must lead to an extremely careful diagnostic reassessment of the patient and should include bronchoscopic sampling of bronchial secretions and haemocultures. In mechanically ventilated pneumonia patients who do not respond to initial therapy the underlying pathogens most likely to be the cause are: *Pseudomonas aeruginosa,* MRSA, *Acinetobacter* spp, *Klebsiella* spp *or Enterobacter* spp. A recent study of VAP patients has indicated that the risk factors linked to therapeutic failure are: older age, duration of mechanical ventilation prior to treatment, presence of neurological disease on admission and no increase of PaO_2/FiO_2 ratio on the third day.

11.6   VAP Prevention Strategies

When confronting VAP it is very important to take appropriate preventive measures.

Generally adopted measures are hand disinfection with alcohol-based gels and the monitoring of invasive devices sites of entry (vascular, endotracheal, gastrointestinal, urinary) in order to maintain their presence at such sites only for the time that proves to be strictly necessary. Intubation and re-intubation increase VAP incidence and, when intubation is necessary, the orotracheal is preferable to the nasotracheal route in order to prevent the onset of sinusitis.

All intensive care units should establish a microbiological monitoring programme for the surveillance of micro-organisms and their resistance over time in order to formulate antibiotic therapies targeted to local flora characteristics and so avoid unnecessary treatments and reduce antibiotic use to the indispensable minimum.

The accumulation of contaminated oropharingeal secretions above the endotracheal cuff adds to the risk of aspiration; removing such excretions lowers the probability of early-onset pneumonia. The cuff filling pressure, a correct value being approximately 20 cmH_2O, should be checked frequently because its perfect adhesion to the tracheal walls ensures minimum pooling of secretions [20].

It is also possible to reduce colonisation and pathogenicity of oropharingeal flora, that was present on admission or was acquired in intensive care, by selective digestive decontamination (SDD) which consists of topical oral antimicrobial agents possibly combined with systemic antimicrobials; many studies have confirmed a reduction of VAP incidence and some studies have also shown reduced mortality [21, 22].

Recent technological development has lead to the manufacture of new endotracheal tubes that have been conceived with a view to reducing bacterial colonisation and biofilm build-up. The tubes are coated with antiseptic layers [23] or with silver [24]. Experimental studies have tested the success of these innovations and have confirmed their effectiveness in reducing both bacterial colonisation and VAP incidence.

Growing evidence has recently endorsed the thesis that patient positioning is crucial in developing VAP and it has been noted that a semirecumbent position may reduce the volume of aspirated secretions when compared to supine position.

Many authors have proven that non-invasive ventilation (NIV) is an effective approach, whether complementary or alternative to invasive ventilation, for selected groups of patients with respiratory failure.

Recommendations for the prevention of VAP are summarised at Table 11.6.

Table 11.6 General recommendations for the prevention of VAP

Hands disinfection with alcohol-based disinfectant
Microbiological surveillance
Monitoring of invasive devices site of entry and early removal
Protocols and plans for the reduction of antibiotic administration
Avoid intubation and re-intubation as far as possible
Select NIV preferably
Select orotracheal tubes and cannulae preferably
Maintain cuff pressure at 20 cmH$_2$O
Prevent tube condensation reflux from entering the airways
Semirecumbent position
Additional measures
Continuous aspiration of sub-glottis secretions
Endotracheal tubes preferably coated with antiseptics or silver
Selective digestive decontamination
Oral decontamination

11.7 Conclusion

Ventilator-associated pneumonia remains a great challenge for the intensivist who must make daily diagnostic and therapeutic decisions that have a direct result on the outcome of critical patients.

Future challenges, besides improvement and widespread use of preventive techniques, include the development of rationalised therapeutic approaches that address the ever increasing problem of antibiotic resistance.

Bibliography

1. Chastre J, Fagon JY (2002) Ventilator-associated pneumonia. Am J Respir Crit Care Med 165:867-903
2. Torres A, Ewig S, Lode H et al. (2009) Defining, treating and preventing hospital acquired pneumonia: European perspective. Intensive Care Med 35:9-29
3. American Thoracic Society (2005) Guidelines for the management of adults with hospital-acquired, ventilator-associated, and healthcare-associated pneumonia. Am J Respir Crit Care Med 171:388-416
4. Fagon JY, Chastre J (2005) Nosocomial pneumonia. In: Fink MP (ed Textbook of critical care, pp 663-677. Elsevier Saunders, Philadelphia
5. Langer M, Cigada M, Mandelli M et al (1987) Early onset pneumonia: a multicenter study in intensive care units. Intensive Care Med 13:342-347
6. Vincent JL, Bihari DJ, Suter PM et al (1995) The prevalence of nosocomial infection in intensive care units in Europe. Results of the European Prevalence of Infection in Intensive Care (EPIC) Study. EPIC international advisory committee. JAMA 274:639-644
7. Cross AS, Roup B (1981) Role of respiratory assistance devices in endemic nosocomial pneumonia. Am J Med 70:681-685
8. Langer M, Mosconi P, Cigada M et al (1989) Long-term respiratory support and risk of pneumonia in critically ill patients. Intensive Care Unit Group of Infection Control. Am Rev Respir Dis 140:302-305
9. Markowicz P, Wolff M, Djedaini K et al (2000) Multicenter prospective study of ventilator associated pneumonia during acute respiratory distress syndrome. Incidence, prognosis and risk factors. ARDS study group. Am J Respir Crit Care Med 161:1942-1948
10. Craven DE (2000) Epidemiology of ventilator-associated pneumonia. Chest 117: 186S-187S
11. Kollef MH, Sherman G, Ward S et al (1999) Inadequate antimicrobial treatment of infections: a risk factor for hospital mortality among critically ill patients. Chest 115: 462-474
12. Rello J, Diaz E, Rodriguez A (2005) Etiology of ventilator-associated pneumonia. Clin Chest Med 26:87-95
13. Park DR (2005) The microbiology of ventilator-associated pneumonia. Respir Care 50:742-763
14. Frutos-Vivar F, Esteban A, Apezteguia C et al (2005) Outcome of mechanically ventilated patients who require a tracheotomy. Crit Care Med 33:290-298
15. Torres A, Ewig S (2004) Diagnosing ventilator-associated pneumonia. N Engl J Med 350:433-435
16. The Canadian Critical Care Trials Group (2006) A randomized trial of diagnostic techniques for ventilator-associated pneumonia. N Engl J Med 355:2619-2629
17. Dupont H, Mentec H, Sollet JP et al (2001) Impact of appropriateness of initial antibiotic therapy on the outcome of ventilator-associated pneumonia. Intensive Care Med 27:355-362
18. Paul M, Soares-Weiser K, Leibovici L (2003) Beta lactam monotherapy versus beta lactam-aminoglycoside combination therapy for fever with neutropenia: systematic review and meta-analysis. BMJ 326:1111-1115
19. Chastre J, Wolff M, Fagon JY et al (2003) Comparison of 8 vs 15 days of antibiotic therapy for ventilator-associated pneumonia in adults: a randomized trial. JAMA 290:2588-2598
20. Cook D, De Jonghe B, Brochard L et al (1998) Influence of airway management on ventilator associated pneumonia: evidence from randomized trials. JAMA 279:781-787
21. Nathens AB, Marshall JC (1999) Selective decontamination of the digestive tract in surgical patients: a systematic review of the evidence. Arch Surg 134:170-176
22. De Smet AMGA, Kluytmans JAJW, Cooper BS et al (2009) Decontamination of the digestive tract and oropharynx in ICU patients. N Engl J Med 360:20-31
23. Berra L, De Marchi L, Yu ZX et al (2004) Endotracheal tube coated with antiseptics decrease bacterial colonization of the ventilatory circuit, lungs and endotracheal tube. Anesthesiology 100:1446-1456
24. Kollef MH, Afessa B, Anzueto A et al (2008) Silver-coated endotracheal tubes and incidence of ventilator associated pneumonia: the NASCENT randomized trial. JAMA 300:805-813

Mechanical Ventilation in Patients with Acute Severe Asthma

12

Davide Chiumello and Sara Sher

12.1 Introduction

The incidence of bronchial asthma is increasing and in the last ten years the associated mortality rate has also risen rapidly. Any doctor may be faced with the treatment of an asthmatic patient under respiratory distress when it becomes necessary to initiate a prompt and aggressive therapy. Starting from epidemiology, pathophysiology and treatment, this chapter deals with the challenge of managing airways and ventilation in case of a severe and acute asthma attack or of status asthmaticus, a term that describes severe and persistent asthma.

12.1.1 Epidemiology

Asthma is the obstruction of the airways; it is variable, it can be completely or partially reversed either spontaneously or through treatment and it is associated to airways inflammation and increased sensitivity to a variety of stimuli. Status asthmaticus is instead progressive respiratory failure due to asthma when it does not respond to conventional treatment with bronchodilating nebulisers [1].

Today asthma is the most common chronic childhood disease with a prevalence of 15-30% in developed countries. There is a great difference in the prevalence of asthma in the world with the highest incidence in UK, Australia and New Zealand and the lowest in Eastern Europe, China and India. Morbidity associated with asthma is also rising. Hospital admissions have doubled in the United Stated in recent years [2]. Europe is following the same

D. Chiumello (✉)
Department of Anesthesiology, Resuscitation and Pain Medicine
Fondazione IRCCS Ca' Granda Ospedale Maggiore Policlinico, Milan, Italy
chiumello@libero.it

Biagio Allaria (ed.), *Practical Issues in Anesthesia and Intensive Care*
© Springer-Verlag Italia 2012

trend. Between 3% and 16% of asthmatic patients admitted to hospital will suffer acute respiratory failure and require intubation and mechanical ventilation [3].

12.1.2 Pathophysiology

Bronchial asthma is characterised by a reversible obstruction of the lower airways caused by local inflammation and oedema, bronchial smooth muscle spasm and mucus plugs [4]. Asthma pathogenesis has lately been deemed to be triggered more by the chronic inflammation of the airways than by bronchial muscle contraction. The level of lymphocytes and eosinophils infiltration found in tracheal and bronchial biopsies of adult asthmatic patients is in fact correlated to the severity of the clinical condition. Epithelial cells, mastocytes and T-lymphocytes are activated and start producing pro-inflammatory cytokines. There is an increase of mediators such as histamine, leukotrienes and platelet-activating factor but, besides the presence of these mediators, it is the destruction of epithelial cells that causes increased irritability of the asthmatic patient's airways [5]. Epithelial cells, especially ciliated cells, are destroyed on the entire length of the trachebronchial tree and nerve endings are therefore exposed. A significant correlation between the extent of damage to epithelial cells and airways' reactivity has been established. Chronically inflamed and hyper-irritable airways are prone to acute obstruction caused by exposure to allergens, by respiratory tract infection, by environmental irritants, by physical exertion, by emotional stress, by gastro-oesophageal reflux, by medication or drug use. Furthermore inflammation causes hypertrophy, stimulates mucous glands and goblet cells and this in turn leads to hypersecretion and, in extreme cases, to the formation of bronchial mucus plugs [6].

12.2 Mechanics of Respiration and Respiratory Function Test (RFT)

The main pathophysiological characteristic of asthma is the narrowed diameter of the airways, a state induced by bronchial smooth muscle contraction, by vascular constriction, by bronchial wall oedema and by thick secretions. The end result is increased expiratory resistance and reduced forced expiratory volume. In fact an asthmatic patient's forced vital capacity (FVC) is ≤ 50% of the normal value; the forced expiratory volume in one second (FEV_1) is 30% of the predicted value and maximum and minimum midexpiratory flow rates are 20% lower than the expected values. In the acute asthma patient the residual volume increases by 400% whereas the functional residual capacity (FRC) doubles. The patient tends to report an improvement and the end of the asthma attack when the residual volume falls to 200% and FEV_1 reaches 50% of the expected value [7].

These altered mechanics of respiration result in air trapping and ensuing pulmonary hyperinflation. Static hyperinflation is caused by premature airways closure during the expiratory phase leading to FRC increase. Dynamic hyperinflation further aggravates the condition since it prevents the patient from completing the expiratory phase before starting the next inspiratory phase. Pulmonary hyperinflation affects respiratory muscles' function, increases respiratory effort and causes respiratory muscle fatigue in the patient [8].

The airways of asthmatic patients close at reduced active expiratory flow, lower speed of gas flow, higher pulmonary volume and closer to the alveoli. The increased airways resistance causes a greater decrease in pressure from the alveoli to the larger bronchi thereby creating the potential for negative intrathoracic transmural pressure (ΔP) and collapsed small airways. In asthma, middle-size airways are narrowed by bronchospasm and if expiration is forced they are further narrowed by negative transmural pressure. The important factor is however the relation between airways closure and FRC; this is what establishes whether any given respiratory section is normal or atelectasic or whether it is a signal of altered ventilation-perfusion ratio (V_A/Q). When the pulmonary volume at which some airways close is greater than tidal volume (VT), the latter does not increase sufficiently during respiration to allow the same airways to open and they remain therefore almost always closed, as in atelectasis. When the closing capacity (CC) of some airways falls within the tidal volume level, the airways will momentarily open as pulmonary volume increases on inspiration and will close again as pulmonary volume decreases on expiration. As these airways are open and closed for a shorter interval than normal airways, they have less time to share in the alveolar gas exchange and this is the equivalent of a reduced V_A/Q. If CC, finally, is lower than all tidal volume respiration, no airway will be closed during the breathing cycle: this is the normal condition. Any factor that causes a decreased FRC in relation to CC or an increased CC in relation to FRC will transform normal respiratory sections into reduced V_A/Q or atelectasic areas thereby causing hypoxaemia [9].

12.3 Cardiopulmonary Interactions

Dynamic hyperinflation in severe asthma leads to significant cardiopulmonary consequences. First of all an increased pulmonary volume results in pulmonary vessels' distension and increased pulmonary vascular resistance with associated right ventricular afterload and a compromise of the right ventricle function. Furthermore such negative intrapleural pressure, on inspiration, leads to increased right venous return that together with increased afterload results in a shift to the left of the intraventricular septum and so in reduced left ventricle filling; the associated elevated afterload due to intrapleural pressure negativity leads to a significant reduction of systolic pressure and output. The exaggerated decline of systolic pressure on inspiration (> 10-12 mmHg) associated to intrapleural pressure variations is called pulsus paradoxus [10].

12.4   Clinical Signs and Diagnostic Picture

12.4.1 General Information

A patient with status asthmaticus generally has a cough, presents signs of dyspnea, of increased respiratory effort and of anxiety. The patient may also present respiratory failure or even cardiopulmonary arrest. Respiratory sounds during auscultation are not related to the seriousness of the patient's condition; on the contrary the plethora of asthmatic sounds in a patient with severe asthma should be reassuring in that they would confirm the presence of albeit the slightest air flow; such minimum flow creates turbulence and vibrations resulting in detectable wheezing. The lack of detectable chest sounds is of much greater concern in the context of increased respiratory effort [11].

12.4.2 Clinical Predictors of Impending Respiratory Failure

The clinical predictors of impending respiratory failure are: altered consciousness, inability to speak, a marked reduction or even absence of respiratory sounds and central cyanosis. Further signs are excessive perspiration and impossibility to assume a supine position [12].

Pulsus paradoxus is an indicator of the asthma attack's seriousness. If the patient's condition allows it and in order to evaluate the asthma attack progression, the extent of pulsus paradoxus can be measured with a simple blood pressure cuff or estimated with a pulse oximeter indicating the trend [13, 14].

Chest X-ray is not indicated in the non-intubated asthmatic patient because radiological anomalies are very seldom found; it is however mandatory when clinical signs and objective examination suggest pneumonia or barotrauma [15].

Haemo-gas analysis provides values on alveolar gas exchange. The early stages of a severe asthma attack reveal hypoxaemia and hypocapnia. As airways obstruction progresses, hypercapnia develops and this is an indicator of imminent respiratory failure. The decision to intubate a patient should however not be based on haemo-gas results but rather on the patient's clinical condition: respiratory effort, pulse oximeter readings and degree of consciousness are correlated clinical indicators of alveolar gas exchange [16]. A sedated and intubated patient requires instead frequent haemo-gas readings, better if obtained by arterial catheter, in order to evaluate ventilation adequacy and to monitor clinical progression [17].

12.5   Treatment and Patient Management

Every status asthmaticus patient requires cardiorespiratory monitoring possibly in a comfortable environment. Even though hypoxaemia and anxiety lead to agitation, sedation is contraindicated in the non-intubated asthmatic patient. The patients admitted to intensive care require venous access, continuous cardiorespiratory monitoring and pulse oximeter use. Patients who breathe spontaneously do not require frequent haemo-gas testing whereas mechanically ventilated patients require a central venous catheter and a Foley catheter [18].

All asthmatic patients suffer from altered ventilation/perfusion ratio and therefore require humidified oxygen that is best administered via non-rebreather mask. If no chronic and persistent lung disease is present, there is no evidence that oxygen may suppress respiratory drive [19].

Asthmatic patients, for the most part, reach medical staff attention in a state of dehydration due to reduced fluid intake, possible vomiting and unnoticed loss of fluids from the respiratory tract. Adequate hydration and maintenance of euvolemic state are necessary to reduce bronchial secretion consistence. Hyperhydration on the contrary is not indicated and could lead to pulmonary oedema because the combination of:
a) increased left ventricle afterload due to negative intrapleural pressure
b) increased capillary permeability caused by pulmonary inflammation promotes transcapillary fluid filtration in the air spaces.

The syndrome of inappropriate antidiuretic hormone (ADH) secretion may be present in severe asthma, therefore a careful monitoring of diuresis and fluid balance must be undertaken [20].

12.5.1 Medication

12.5.1.1 β-agonists

β-receptors agonist bronchodilators are essential in the treatment of status asthmaticus. They mediate bronchodilation by stimulating β_2-receptors on the bronchial smooth muscle.

The most commonly used agents are adrenaline, isoproterenol, terbutaline and salbutamol. Terbutaline and salbutamol are generally the preferred choice for their β_2-selective action hence the lower probability of a β_1 effect on cardiovascular receptors.

β-agonists may be administered through inhalation, IV, subcutaneously or orally but the most used method is nebulisation. The most used drug is salbutamol at a suggested dosage of 0.05 up to 0.15 mg/kg. The correct dose is not well defined but it has been observed that even in ideal conditions less than 10% of the drug reaches the lungs; lately much higher doses have therefore been suggested. Respiratory volumes and pattern and nebuliser flow further cause variations to the quantity of medication that actually reaches its site of action. Continuous nebulisation is preferable to intermittent administration. Most studies report the use of nebulised salbutamol at fairly low dosage (4-10 mg/h) but much higher doses have also been mentioned up to its use in undiluted and nebulised form (150 mg/h with 10-12 L/min flow). Nebulisation, regardless of the method of administration, must always include oxygen.

If a patient does not respond to continuous nebulisation, IV *β-agonists* should be considered. A reduction in tidal volume and/or almost complete obstruction during severe status asthmaticus may prevent nebulised medication to reach the most affected areas. Salbutamol remains the most commonly employed drug at a dosage ranging from 0.5 up to 5 μg/kg/min.

The major side effects of this drug are of cardiovascular nature. Tachycardia, prolonged QTc interval, arrhythmia, hypertension and hypotension have been reported both with IV and inhalation administration; neither salbutamol nor terbutaline, however, cause significant cardiotoxicity except for tachycardia and diastolic hypotension in status asthmaticus patients. Cardiac ischaemia is instead a possible complication of IV isoprotenerol. Other side effects of β-agonist drugs are hypokalaemia, tremor and deterioration of ventilation/perfusion ratio. Adverse effects of cardiovascular nature reveal tachyphylaxis but not bronchodilation. Long-acting $β_2$-agonists, such as salmeterol, are contraindicated in status asthmaticus since in this context they have been linked to mortality [21, 17].

Hypokalaemia and hyperglicaemia are the most common metabolic side effects; treatment is not usually necessary but levels should be monitored during treatment with inhaled β-agonists and a further administration of potassium, in addition to the maintenance dose, may be required [18].

12.5.1.2 Corticosteroids

Inflammation is at the base of asthma pathophysiology and treatment is therefore based on corticosteroids both in an acute attack and in chronic asthma [22]. Some of the many effects of corticosteroids are: suppression of cytokines production, suppression of granulocyte macrophage colony-stimulating factor (GM-CSF) and suppression of inducible nitric oxide synthase all of which are inflammatory process mediators in asthma. Corticosteroids immunosuppressive action prevents recruitment and activation of inflammatory cells, reduces mucus production and reduces microvascular permeability.

Systemic administration of corticosteroids lowers the rate of hospital admissions and also the duration of hospital stay whereas inhaled dosing is not indicated in the acute attack. The most used agent is methylprednisolone by virtue of its limited mineralcorticoid effects. The initial IV dose is 2 mg/kg followed by 0.5-1 mg/kg every 6 hours. Corticosteroids effect begins after 1-3 hours and peaks after 4-8 hours. Treatment duration depends on the severity of the condition but administration is usually continued until case resolution [23]. Prolonged use may lead to the suppression of the hypothalamic-pituitary-adrenal axis, to osteoporosis, myopathy and muscle weakness, the last two complications worsen with the concurrent administration of neuromuscular blocking drugs in patients under invasive mechanical ventilation [18].

12.5.1.3 Anticholinergics

The anticholinergic agent mostly used during an asthma attack is ipratropium bromide. It promotes bronchodilation without inhibiting mucociliary clearance as instead is the case with atropine. Nebulised ipratropium bromide acts as a sympathetic cholinergic blocking agent and antagonizes acethylcholine by blocking its interaction with muscarinic receptors on the bronchial smooth muscle cells so that intracellular levels of cyclic guanosine monophosphate (cGMP) are reduced and muscle contraction is prevented. Ipratropium bromide, when administered in the emergency department, lowers both the rate of hospital admissions and the index of asthma attacks' severity. This drug, when compared to β-agonists and corticosteroids, does not however offer any further clinical advantages to the patient already in hospital; the majority of authors nevertheless supports its administration in nebulised form in critical patients who do not respond to aggressive treatment. Ipratropium bromide has few side effects by virtue of its minimal systemic absorption; the most common are dry mouth, flushing, tachycardia and vertigo [18].

12.5.2 Intubation

12.5.2.1 Indications and Intubation Methods
The decision to intubate an asthmatic patient should never be acted upon in an emergency situation. Tracheal intubation may aggravate bronchospasm and positive pressure ventilation may considerably increase the risk of barotrauma and of circulatory depression. Respiratory acidosis is not an indication for intubation whereas intubation is indicated in respiratory and cardiac arrest, severe hypoxia and fast deterioration of consciousness. Progressive respiratory fatigue, despite maximum treatment, is also a relative indication for mechanical ventilation. In all other cases, every severely asthmatic patient should receive an aggressive treatment with nebulised β2-agonists, anticholinergics and corticosteroids. The decision to intubate should not be based on haemogas levels since some hypercapnic patients can be successfully treated also without mechanical ventilation whereas some others who have reached the point of exhaustion need to be intubated whether they are hypercapnic or not [17].

Tracheal intubation of a patient with status asthmaticus is a very delicate manoeuvre that should be carried out by the most experienced anaesthetist-reanimator and, if possible, not unassisted [18].

The patient must be pre-oxygenated with 100% oxygen, oropharingeal secretions must be aspirated and the stomach emptied via nasogastric tube. Premedication with a sedative or anaesthetic should always be conducted and then followed by administration of a hypnotic/sedative drug and of a fast-acting myorelaxant drug. Neuromuscular block prevents broad variations of pressure in the airways, variations that are instead present after intubation in an asthmatic patient who has not received curare. The choice must fall on a cuffed tracheal tube of the greatest possible diameter in order to reduce the already high resistance an asthmatic patient has [24].

After pre-oxygenation, orotracheal rapid sequence intubation is carried out. This method lowers the risk of gastric content aspiration. Afterwards it is possible to proceed to a replacement with a nasotracheal tube, which is better tolerated especially by children.

Of all complications that arise in the asthmatic patient in need of intubation, over 50% actually start during or immediately after intubation. Complications, besides tube malpositioning, are secondary to air trapping and include hypotension, cardiac arrest, de-saturation and pneumothorax with subcutaneous emphysema [25, 26]. Exhaled CO_2 monitoring is mandatory as it will confirm correct positioning of the endotracheal tube. The tube's obstruction caused by very thick bronchial secretions sometimes requires tube replacement. Arterial hypotension is not rare after the asthmatic patient is intubated and it is caused by hyperinflation and consequent decrease of venous return to the heart combined with the cardiodepressant and vasodilating effect of hypnotic and neuromuscular blocking agents. Hyperinflation usually responds to fluid administration and to respiratory rate reduction; the extent of hyperinflation contribution to hypotension can in fact be determined by observing pressure response to an abrupt reduction of respiratory rate or even to a period of apnoea.

In some severely asthmatic patients, manual pressure applied to the rib cage during expiration may become necessary in order to avoid massive hyperinflation. When hypotension and/or hypoxaemia do not respond to either fluids administration or to the change of ventilation pattern, possible pneumothorax must be considered [17, 26].

12.5.2.2 Induction and Intubation Medications

Ketamine is a dissociative anaesthetic with a potent analgesic effect. It causes bronchodilation but the mechanism is not yet well understood; its action is sympathomimetic and inhibits noradrenaline neuronal reuptake; it also appears to block N-metil-D-aspartate receptors which are linked to increased muscular tone of the airways. Ketamine is mostly used in severely asthmatic children under mechanical ventilation because of its anaesthetic and bronchodilating properties. Administration starts with IV bolus of 2 mg/kg followed by continuous infusion of 0.5-2 mg/kg/h. Ketamine is a very useful induction agent for ventilation since it reduces bronchial constriction response when the tube is inserted in the airways and it also maintains haemodynamic stability at this delicate stage. Undesirable side effects of ketamine are increased bronchial secretions (so it should be administered together with atropine) and its capability to cause visual hallucinations especially in adult patients. Its indirect sympathomimetic effect prompts cardiac hyperdynamic response but could also have a cardiodepressant effect in the critical patient who lacks catecholaminergic reserves. Ketamine also increases cerebral blood flow through vasodilation and should therefore be used with care in those patients at risk of endocranial hypertension such as patients with previous hypoxic-ischaemic injury or with severe hypercapnia [27].

Inhalation anaesthetics have for some time been used in the treatment of irresponsive status asthmaticus [28]. Their precise mechanism of action remains unclear. Halothane and isoflurane have been successfully employed in mechanically ventilated patients with severe asthma who did not respond to other treatments [29]. The correct and safe administration of such agents requires an anaesthesia machine or an adapted ventilator and continuous testing of inspired and expired gas. Possible adverse effects of halothane are arrhythmia-inducing cardiodepressant action especially when hypoxia is present, acidosis and hypercapnia when used in combination with β-agonists or aminophylline. Isoflurane does not have a cardiodepressant action nor does it cause arrhythmia but it may induce hypotension as a consequence of peripheral vasodilation. Inhalation anaesthetics may aggravate shunting due to suppression of the hypoxic pulmonary vasoconstriction mechanism. As there is no significant difference in the bronchodilating effect of either one or the other anaesthetic, isoflurane remains the safest choice [17].

12.5.2.3 Sedation and Neuromuscular Block
The hypercapnic patient under mechanical ventilation requires sedation in order to avoid tachypnoea and loss of synchronization with the ventilator. Continuous infusion of benzodiazepines such as midazolam or lorazepam may be used, or also fentanyl. Morphine should be avoided due to its capability to release histamine. Ketamine, by virtue of its bronchodilating effect remains the best choice.

Neuromuscular block should be limited to patients for whom it is not possible to achieve adequate ventilation at acceptable inspiratory pressure. Avoiding neuromuscular block lowers the risk of potential neuromuscular complications. Prolonged muscle weakness has in fact been reported in patients who in the course of mechanical ventilation received steroids and neuromuscular blocking agents. In this acute myopathy there are rhabdomyolysis signs, such as an increased creatine phosphokinase level and myonecrosis in muscle biopsies [30, 31]. It is a reversible but prolonged myopathy and even if its onset cannot be ascribed with certainty to neuromuscular blocking agents, it is recommended to limit both their dosage and the duration of use [17].

12.5.3 Mechanical Ventilation (Table 12.1)

12.5.3.1 Dynamic Hyperinflation
Positive pressure ventilation greatly alters cardiocirculatory and respiratory dynamics in the asthmatic patient. Intrapleural pressure changes from negative to positive prompting venous return reduction, hence hypotension. Hypotension will respond to fluid infusion and respiratory rate reduction.

The severe obstruction of air flow results in incomplete expiration even before intubation and this leads to dynamic hyperinflation with end expiration volume exceeding functional residual capacity. The increased pulmonary volume boosts the strength of pulmonary elastic recoil thus increasing expiratory flow; it also causes small airways to expand thus reducing expiratory resistance. For this reason pulmonary volume will increase up to the point when the entire inspired tidal volume will be expired within the available time. In severe asthma however, this process fails to adapt and so the level of hyperinflation that is necessary to maintain normocapnia cannot be achieved since it would exceed total lung capacity. Once positive pressure ventilation is established, the degree of dynamic hyperinflation correlates to the set tidal volume and to the expiratory time and also to the extent of airways obstruction. Conventional methods of ventilation targeted at normocapnia typically lead to dynamic hyperinflation with increased risk of hypotension and barotrauma [32, 17].

In severe asthma, the level of dynamic hyperinflation must be constantly monitored in order to identify those patients with severe dynamic hyperinflation who could be at risk of complications and also to evaluate airways obstruction progression. Two are the methods: measuring total expiratory flow during prolonged apnoea, starting at the end of inspiration, and evaluating airways pressure during volume-controlled ventilation. The pressure to be measured is the plateau pressure (Pplat) because it is not affected by flow-resistance properties. An increased Pplat is usually a sign of dynamic hyperinflation since patients with airways obstruction typically have respiratory system compliance. Although a precise Pplat value that would increase barotrauma risk has not been established, a maximum of 25-30 cmH_2O is generally accepted [33, 24].

Table 12.1 Mechanical ventilation in severe asthma

Ventilator Settings	
Modality	Assist-control
Tidal volume	8-9 mL/kg
Respiratory frequency	12-14 breaths/min
Minute ventilation	0.1-0.13 L/kg/min
Inspiratory flow	60-70 L/min
Wave shape	decelerating or square
PEEP	≤ 5 cmH_2O
%FiO_2	$SatO_2 > 90\%$
Sedation and blockade	
Propofol	2.5 mg/kg/h infusion
Fentanyl	50-200 mcg/h infusion
Vecuronium	0.1 mg/kg bolus
Treatment of obstructed airways	
Salbutamol-ipratropium	6 puff qh x 4, then q1-2h
Methylprednisolone	1-2 mg/kg/die
Ventilator settings adjustments	

Target: Pplat < 30 cmH_2O (≤25 ideal) and pH ≥7.2
- Pplat > 30 cmH_2O → reduce minute ventilation
- pH < 7.2 e Pplat < 25 → increase minute ventilation
- pH < 7.2 e Pplat 25-30 → do not change (consider bicarbonate in case of unstable haemodynamics)

12.5.3.2 Permissive Hypercapnia

The main purpose of mechanical ventilation in status asthmaticus is to provide adequate oxygenation and minimise the risk of barotrauma. As barotrauma risk is linked to dynamic lung hyperinflation and to high plateau pressure, the ventilation strategy must be targeted at minimising pulmonary volume and airways pressure. The currently adopted system of mechanical ventilation in status asthmaticus is controlled hypoventilation. This method enables PCO2 to increase for as long as minute ventilation and the fraction of inspired oxygen (FiO_2) are sufficient to maintain adequate tissue oxygenation. The acceptance of hypercapnia in this context is defined as permissible hypercapnia. The reason for this approach is that hypercapnia carries a lesser risk when compared to that of a greatly increased pulmonary volume [34, 35].

Physiological response to respiratory and metabolic acidosis includes increased cardiac output, pulmonary pressure and heart rate while systemic vascular resistance decreases and systemic arterial pressure remains stable. These changes in haemodynamics are mediated by endogenous catecholamines that are stimulated by a decreased blood pH. In this instance, bicarbonate infusion reduces acidosis thus worsening haemodynamic balance and proving not to be useful in increasing bronchodilation or survival. Furthermore, since bicarbonate reacts to hydrogen ions by producing CO2, this molecule's levels increase and CO_2 disperses in the cells causing paradoxical intracellular acidosis thereby worsening the mortality rate. For these reasons bicarbonate infusion is only recommended when acidosis has significant haemodynamic relevance. The minimum safe pH level during permissive hypercapnia is not known [35]. The most serious complications of hypercapnia are increased cerebral blood flow and intracranial pressure especially in patients who have suffered anoxic damage secondary to respiratory arrest prior to intubation [33].

12.5.3.3 Initial Ventilator Settings

The most adequate mechanical ventilation may vary from patient to patient and it also depends on the disease stage. Most doctors prefer pressure controlled ventilation as the initial setup. Because of decelerating flow patterns, pressure controlled ventilation or pressure control with volume guarantee (PC-VG) will result in reduced peak pressure but higher mean pressure of airways in relation to the same tidal volume administered in volume controlled ventilation mode. Inspiratory time must be set up at 0.75-1.5 seconds. Peak pressure is likely to be elevated in patients with severe asthma because of the elevated inspiratory flow added to severe airways obstruction. For this reason peak pressure is not representative of alveolar pressure and is therefore not as reliable an indicator as plateau pressure to determine barotrauma risk. Despite this and considering the different areas of airway obstruction, it is possible for some distal airways to be directly exposed to elevated proximal pressure and so to be at risk of barotrauma. It is therefore necessary to try and maintain inspiratory peak pressure below 40 cmH2O [17].

Administration of neuromuscular blocking agents is often necessary in order to maintain low airway pressure during mechanical ventilation.

The use of positive end-expiratory pressure (PEEP) in the asthmatic patient under mechanical ventilation remains a debated subject. Some authors advise against its use since it would increase air-trapping. On the other hand a low PEEP may reduce airways dynamic collapse in asthma and lessen the trigger effort of ventilated patients with spontaneous respiration [36, 37]. In the asthmatic patient, PEEP should in any case be set at a lower value than auto-PEEP and measured by the expiratory pause method in order to lessen trigger effort without preventing expiratory flow [17, 18, 24].

12.5.3.4 Ventilator Settings Adjustments

Setting hypoventilation mode will lead to hypercapnia which is well tolerated, even when extreme, provided there is no increased intracranial pressure and that pH is not above 7.10, a level usually tolerated as long as oxygenation is good (oxygen > 90% with FiO_2 < 0.6). Expiratory time adequacy may be evaluated by listening for the end of wheezing before the next respiratory action starts and by observing a return to baseline values on the flow-time curve or alternatively by observing plateau pressure on the curve of exhaled CO_2. It will be difficult, initially, to reach such targets but as the airways obstruction improves the curves will stabilise and the reduction of both peak and plateau pressure will indicate an improvement of respiratory diynamics.

Return to spontaneous respiration must be enabled by switching to a different ventilation mode. PC and VGPR are pressure control modes where each action that the patient triggers, as well as those already set up on the ventilator, are delivered at pre-set pressure or volume values. In the dyspnoic and agitated patient this leads to a worsening of hyperinflation. For this reason, once neuro-muscular block and sedation are withdrawn to allow spontaneous respiration, the ventilator should be re-set to synchronized intermittent mandatory ventilation (SIMV) mode with pressure support (PS) or to pressure support mode only. This enables the patient to achieve his/her respiratory pattern (frequency, inspiratory time, tidal volume), it reduces patient-ventilator asynchrony and respiratory effort by totally or at least partially assisting the respiratory muscles [38].

Pressure support ventilation may also be set immediately after intubation when the asthmatic patient requires complete and total support. There have been case reports of fast improvement in patients' alveolar gas exchange, inspiratory pressure and respiratory mechanics after switching the patients from pressure controlled ventilation to elevated pressure support (22-37 cmH_2O). With this method not only is the inspiratory effort reduced but the patient has the possibility to actively sustain expiration thus reducing hyperinflation [17].

12.6   Conclusion

Status asthmaticus is a medical emergency that any doctor may have to face especially when considering the growing incidence of asthma in the Western world population. Knowledge of the correct management of both medical treatment and ventilation support and of possible complications mainly linked to increased airways resistance and consequently to dynamic pulmonary hyperinflation is essential in order to improve the management of these patients and their mortality rate.

Bibliography

1. Albert R, Slutsky A, Ranieri M et al (2006) Clinical critical care medicine. Elsevier, Philadelphia
2. Sly RM (1999) Changing prevalence of allergic rhinitis and asthma. Ann Asthma Allergy Immunology 82:233-248
3. Santiago SM, Klaustermeyer WB (1980) Mortality in status asthmaticus: nine-year experience in a respiratory ICU. J Asthma Res 17:75-79
4. Cerveri I, Corsico AG (2009) What defines air flow obstruction in asthma? Eur Respir J 34:3
5. Chung KF (1999) Non-invasive biomarkers of asthma. Pediatric Pulmonol Supp 18:41-44
6. Latinen LA, Heino M, Latinen A et al (1985) Damage of airway epithelium and bronchial reactivity in patients with asthma. Am Rev Respir Dis 131:599-606
7. Harrison's Principles of internal medicine (2001) 15th ed. McGraw-Hill, New York
8. Cormier Y, Lecours R, Legris C (1990) Mechanisms of hyperinflation in asthma. Eur Respir J 3:619-624
9. Miller's Anesthesia (2005) 6th ed. Elsevier Churchill Livingston, Philadelphia
10. Rebuck AS, Pengelly LD (1973) Development of pulsus paradoxus in the presence of airway obstruction. N Engl J Med 288:66-69
11. McFadden ER J, Kiser R, DeGroot WJ (1973) Acute bronchial asthma: relation between clinical and physiologic manifestations. N Engl J Med 288:221-225
12. Brenner B, Abraham E, Simon R (1983) Position and diaphoresis in acute asthma. Am J Med 74:1005-1009
13. Wright RO, Steele DW, Santucci KA et al (1996) Continuous, non-invasive measurement of pulsus paradoxus in patients with acute asthma. Arch Pediatr Adolesc Med 150:914-918
14. National Asthma Education and Prevention Program (1997) Expert panel report 2: Guidelines for the diagnosis and management of asthma. NIH Publication No. 55-4015
15. Brooks LJ, Cloutier MM, Afshani E (1982) Significance of roentgenographic abnormalities in children hospitalized for asthma. Chest 82:315-318
16. Weiss EB, Faling LJ (1968) Clinical significance of PaCO2 during status asthmaticus: the crossover point. Ann Allergy 26:545-551
17. Werner HA (2001) Status asthmaticus in children: a review Chest 119:1913-1929
18. Roger's Textbook of pediatric intensive care (2008) Lippicnott Williams & Wilkins, Philadelphia
19. Schiff M (1980) Control of breathing in asthma. Clin Chest Med 1:85-89
20. Baker JW, Yerger S, Segar WE (1976) Elevated plasma antidiuretic hormone levels in status asthmaticus. Mayo Clinic Proc 51:31-34
21. DeNicola LK, Monem GF, Gayle MO et al (1994) Treatment of critical status asthmaticus in children. Pediatr Clinic North Am 41:1293-1324
22. Barnes PJ (1990) Effect of corticosteroids on airway hyperresponsiveness. Am Rev Respir Dis 141:S70-S76
23. Warner JO, Naspitz CK (1998) Third International Pediatric Consensus statement on the management of childhood asthma: International Pediatric Asthma Consensus Group. Pediatr Pulmonol 25:1-17
24. Cox RG, Barker GA, Bohn DJ (1991) Efficacy, results and complications of mechanical ventilation in children with status asthmaticus. Pediatr Pulmonol 11:120-126
25. Zimmerman JL, Dellinger RP, Shah AN et al (1993) Endotracheal intubation and mechanical ventilation in severe asthma. Crit Care Med 21:1727-1730

26. Tuxen DV, Lane S (1987) The effects of ventilatory pattern on hyperinflation, airway pressures, and circulation in mechanical ventilation of patients with severe airflow obstruction. Am Rev Resp Dis 136:872-879
27. L'Hommedieu CS, Arens JJ (1987) The use of ketamine for the emergency intubation of patients with status asthmaticus. Ann Emerg Med 16:568-571
28. Mytum CK (1931) Bronchial asthma: relief of prolonged attack by administration of ether. Med Clin North Am 15:201-210
29. Johnston RG, Noseworthy TW, Friesen EG et al (1990) Isoflurane therapy for status asthmaticus in children and adults. Chest 97:698-701
30. Douglas JA, Tuxen DV, Horne M (1992) Myopathy in severe asthma. Am Rev Respir Dis 146:517-519
31. Leatherman JW, Fleugel WW, David WD et al (1966) Muscle weakness in asthmatic patients who undergo mechanical ventilation. Am J Respir Crit Care Med 153:1686-1690
32. Leatherman JW, McArthur C, Shapiro RS (2004) Effect of prolongation of expiratory time on dynamic hyperinflation in mechanically ventilated patients with severe asthma. Crit Care Med 32:1542-1545
33. Tobin M (2006) Principles and practice of mechanical ventilation, 2nd ed. McGrawHill
34. Darioli R, Perret C (1984) Mechanical controlled hypoventilation in status asthmaticus. Am Rev Respir Dis 129:385
35. Irwin RS, Rippe JM (2008) Irwin and Rippe's Intensive Care Medicine. Lippincott Williams & Wilkins, 6th ed
36. Smith TC, Marini JJ (1988) Impact of PEEP on lung mechanics and work of breathing in severe airflow obstruction. J Appl Physiol 65:1488-1499
37. Tan IK, Bhatt SB, Tam YH et al (1993) Effects of PEEP on dynamic hyperinflation in patients with airflow limitation. Br J Anaesth 70:267-272
38. Wetzel RC (1996) Pressure support ventilation in children with severe asthma. Crit Care Med 24:1603-1605